Health Equity in Endocrinology

Editors

SHERITA HILL GOLDEN
RANA MALEK

ENDOCRINOLOGY AND METABOLISM CLINICS OF NORTH AMERICA

www.endo.theclinics.com

Consulting Editor
ROBERT RAPAPORT

December 2023 • Volume 52 • Number 4

ELSEVIER

1600 John F. Kennedy Boulevard • Suite 1800 • Philadelphia, Pennsylvania, 19103-2899

http://www.theclinics.com

ENDOCRINOLOGY AND METABOLISM CLINICS OF NORTH AMERICA Volume 52, Number 4
December 2023 ISSN 0889-8529, ISBN 13: 978-0-443-18364-5

Editor: Taylor Hayes
Developmental Editor: Saswoti Nath

Endocrinology and Metabolism Clinics of North America (ISSN 0889-8529) is published quarterly by Elsevier Inc., 360 Park Avenue South, New York, NY 10010-1710. Months of issue are March, June, September, and December. Periodicals postage paid at New York, NY and additional mailing offices. Subscription prices are USD 406.00 per year for US individuals, USD 907.00 per year for US institutions, USD 100.00 per year for US students and residents, USD 481.00 per year for Canadian individuals, USD 1121.00 per year for Canadian institutions, USD 527.00 per year for international individuals, USD 1121.00 per year for international institutions, USD 100.00 per year for Canadian students/residents, and USD 245.00 per year for international students/residents. To receive student/resident rate, orders must be accompanied by name of affiliated institution, date of term, and the signature of program/residency coordinator on institution letterhead. Orders will be billed at individual rate until proof of status is received. Foreign air speed delivery is included in all *Clinics* subscription prices. All prices are subject to change without notice. **POSTMASTER:** Send address changes to *Endocrinology and Metabolism Clinics of North America*, Elsevier Health Sciences Division, Subscription Customer Service, 3251 Riverport Lane, Maryland Heights, MO 63043. **Customer Service: Telephone: 1-800-654-2452** (U.S. and Canada); **1-314-447-8871** (outside U.S. and Canada). **Fax: 1-314-447-8029. E-mail: journalscustomerservice-usa@elsevier.com (for print support)**; **journalsonlinesupport-usa@elsevier.com (for online support)**.

Reprints. For copies of 100 or more, of articles in this publication, please contact the Commercial Rights Department, Elsevier Inc., 360 Park Avenue South, New York, NY 10010-1710; phone: +1-212-633-3874; fax: +1-212-633-3820; E-mail: reprints@elsevier.com.

Endocrinology and Metabolism Clinics of North America is covered in *MEDLINE/PubMed (Index Medicus), EMBASE/Excerpta Medica, Current Contents/Clinical Medicine, Current Contents/Life Sciences, Science Citation Index, ISI/BIOMED, BIOSIS,* and *Chemical Abstracts*.

Contributors

CONSULTING EDITOR

ROBERT RAPAPORT, MD
Professor of Pediatrics, Emma Elizabeth Sullivan Professor of Pediatric Endocrinology and Diabetes, Icahn School of Medicine at Mount Sinai, Director, Emeritus, Division of Pediatric Endocrinology and Diabetes Kravis Children's Hospital at Mount Sinai, New York, New York, USA

EDITORS

SHERITA HILL GOLDEN, MD, MHS
Professor, Vice President, and Chief Diversity Officer, Johns Hopkins Medicine, Division of Endocrinology, Diabetes, and Metabolism, Johns Hopkins School of Medicine, Baltimore, Maryland, USA

RANA MALEK, MD
Associate Professor of Medicine, University of Maryland School of Medicine, Baltimore, Maryland, USA

AUTHORS

SHARL S. AZAR, MD
Medical Director, Comprehensive Sickle Cell Disease Treatment Center, Hematology and Medical Oncology Division, Department of Medicine, Massachusetts General Hospital, Harvard Medical School, Boston, Massachusetts, USA

GABRIELA BEROUKHIM, MD
Resident, Department of Obstetrics, Gynecology, and Reproductive Sciences, Yale School of Medicine, New Haven, Connecticut, USA

KEVIN J. BODE PADRON, BS
Medical Student, Duke University School of Medicine, Massachusetts General Hospital Neuroendocrine and Pituitary Tumor Clinical Center, Boston, Massachusetts, USA

NICHOLA Z. BOMANI, BA
Medical Student, Massachusetts General Hospital Neuroendocrine and Pituitary Tumor Clinical Center, Case Western Reserve University School of Medicine, Boston, Massachusetts, USA

LINETTE BOSQUES, MD, PhD
Internal Medicine Resident, Department of Medicine, Massachusetts General Hospital, Harvard Medical School, Boston, Massachusetts, USA

PHILIPPA BOULLE, MBBS, MPH, DHTM
Médecins Sans Frontières Doctors without Borders, Geneva, Switzerland

SHERRI-ANN M. BURNETT-BOWIE, MD, MPH
Associate Professor of Medicine, Endocrine Division, Department of Medicine, Massachusetts General Hospital, Harvard Medical School, Boston, Massachusetts, USA

SARA J. CROMER, MD
Assistant in Medicine, Endocrine Division, Department of Medicine, Massachusetts General Hospital, Harvard Medical School, Boston, Massachusetts, USA

ALICIA DIAZ-THOMAS, MD, MPH
Professor of Pediatrics, Associate Dean of Faculty Affairs, Pediatric Endocrinology Fellowship Program Director, Department of Pediatrics, Division of Pediatric Endocrinology, The University of Tennessee Health Science Center, Memphis, Tennessee, USA

SANDRA ECHEVERRIA, PhD
Associate Professor, Department of Public Health Education, Greensboro, North Carolina, USA

DEBORAH A. ELLIS, PhD
Professor, Department of Family Medicine and Public Health Sciences, Wayne State University School of Medicine, Detroit, Michigan, USA

TOM ELLMAN, MBChB, MRCP
Médecins Sans Frontières Doctors without Borders, Marshalltown, Johannesburg, South Africa

TERRY P. GAO, MD
Department of General Surgery, Temple University Hospital, Philadelphia, Pennsylvania, USA

JASHALYNN C. GERMAN, MD
Fellow, Duke University School of Medicine, Massachusetts General Hospital Neuroendocrine and Pituitary Tumor Clinical Center, Boston, Massachusetts, USA

APOORVA GOMBER, MBBS, MD, MPH
Associate Director of Advocacy, Division of Global Health Equity, Brigham and Women's Hospital, Center for Integration Science, Boston, Massachusetts, USA

REBECCA L. GREEN, MD
Resident, Department of General Surgery, Temple University Hospital, Philadelphia, Pennsylvania, USA

ADRIANA G. IOACHIMESCU, MD, PhD
Professor of Medicine (Endocrinology and Molecular Medicine) and Neurosurgery, Medical College of Wisconsin, HUB for Collaborative Medicine, Milwaukee, Wisconsin, USA

PALLAVI IYER, MD
Associate Professor of Pediatrics, Section Chief and Medical Director Pediatric Endocrinology, Department of Pediatrics, Section of Pediatric Endocrinology, Medical College of Wisconsin, Children's Corporate Center, Milwaukee, Wisconsin, USA

KIRAN JOBANPUTRA, MBChB, MPH
Médecins Sans Frontières, Chancery Exchange, London, United Kingdom

JOSHUA J. JOSEPH, MD, MPH, FAHA
Associate Professor of Internal Medicine, Division of Endocrinology, Diabetes and Metabolism, The Ohio State University College of Medicine, Columbus, Ohio, USA

SYLVIA KEHLENBRINK, MD
Director, Global Endocrinology, Division of Endocrinology, Diabetes and Metabolism, Brigham and Women's Hospital, Boston, Massachusetts, USA

KARLA N. KENDRICK, MD, MPH
Obesity Medicine Physician, Beth Israel Lahey Health, Winchester Hospital Weight Management Center, Winchester, Massachusetts, USA

LINDSAY E. KUO, MD, MBA
Assistant Professor of Surgery, Department of General Surgery, Temple University Hospital, Philadelphia, Pennsylvania, USA

LENNY LÓPEZ, MD, MPH, MDiv, FAHA
Professor of Medicine, University of California, San Francisco, San Francisco VA Medical Center, San Francisco, California, USA

ELIZABETH LAMOS, MD
Associate Professor of Medicine, University of Maryland School of Medicine, Baltimore, Maryland, USA

IRVING LING, MD
Community Medicine and Urban Health Fellow, Kaiser Permanente Northern California, San Francisco, California, USA

LAUREN Y. MALDONADO, MD, MPH
Resident Physician, Department of Medicine, Massachusetts General Hospital and Harvard Medical School, Department of Pediatrics, MassGeneral Hospital for Children and Harvard Medical School, Boston, Massachusetts, USA

RANA MALEK, MD
Associate Professor of Medicine, University of Maryland School of Medicine, Baltimore, Maryland, USA

SYLVIE NAAR, PhD
Distinguished Endowed Professor, Center for Translational Behavioral Medicine, Florida State University, Tallahassee, Florida, USA

ANNA T. NAKAYAMA, MSc, RD, LDN, ANutr
International Alliance for Diabetes Action, St Louis, Missouri, USA

RACHEL NUGENT, PhD
Associate Professor, Department of Global Health, University of Washington, Seattle, Washington, USA

DENNIS D. NYANYO, BA
Medical Student, Massachusetts General Hospital Neuroendocrine and Pituitary Tumor Clinical Center, Harvard Medical School, Harvard Kennedy School of Government, Boston, Massachusetts, USA

AMULYA REDDY, MD, MPH
Médecins Sans Frontières, Chancery Exchange, London, United Kingdom

ROBERT M. SARGIS, MD, PhD
Associate Professor, College of Medicine, Division of Endocrinology, Diabetes, and Metabolism, University of Illinois at Chicago, Chicago Center for Health and Environment, Section of Endocrinology, Diabetes, and Metabolism, Jesse Brown Veterans Affairs Medical Center, Chicago, Illinois, USA

MAURO SARMIENTO, MD, PhD
Statewide Medical Director–Maryland, YesCare Corporation, Hanover, Maryland, USA

DAVID B. SEIFER, MD
Professor, Department of Obstetrics, Gynecology, and Reproductive Sciences, Yale School of Medicine, New Haven, Connecticut, USA

FATIMA CODY STANFORD, MD, MPH, MPA, MBA
Associate Professor of Medicine and Pediatrics, Harvard Medical School, Obesity Medicine Physician-Scientist, Massachusetts General Hospital, Boston, Massachusetts, USA

LUCY TU
Undergraduate Student, Departments of Sociology and History of Science, Harvard University, Cambridge, Massachusetts, USA

VINOD VARMA, MD, MA
The Global Fund to Fight AIDS, Tuberculosis and Malaria, Geneva, Switzerland

BRENDA VARRIANO, MD, MSc
Resident, Central Michigan College of Medicine, Mount Pleasant, Michigan, USA

LUYU WANG, BS
MD/PhD Student, College of Medicine, Division of Endocrinology, Diabetes, and Metabolism, University of Illinois at Chicago, Chicago, Illinois, USA

MARGARET C. WEISS, BS
MD/PhD Student, School of Public Health, College of Medicine, Division of Endocrinology, Diabetes, and Metabolism, University of Illinois at Chicago, Chicago, Illinois, USA

ELAINE W. YU, MD, MMSc
Endocrine Division, Department of Medicine, Massachusetts General Hospital, Assistant Professor, Harvard Medical School, Boston, Massachusetts, USA

RUTH ENID ZAMBRANA, PhD
Professor, Harriet Tubman Department of Women, Gender and Sexuality Studies, Distinguished University Professor, University of Maryland, Director, Consortium on Race, Gender and Ethnicity, College Park, Maryland, USA

Contents

Foreword: Disparities in Endocrinology Care xiii

Robert Rapaport

Preface: Recognizing and Addressing Health Inequities in Endocrinology and Diabetes xv

Sherita Hill Golden and Rana Malek

Advancing Equity in Diabetes Prevention, Treatment, and Outcomes: Delivering on Our Values 559

Joshua J. Joseph

Diabetes inequities exist from diabetes prevention to outcomes and are rooted in the social drivers (determinants) of health. Historical policies such as "redlining" have adversely affected diabetes prevalence, control, and outcomes for decades. Advancing diabetes equity requires multimodal approaches, addressing both individual-level diabetes education, self-management, and treatment along with addressing social needs, and working to improve upstream drivers of health. All individuals affected by diabetes must advocate for policies to advance diabetes equity at the organizational, local, state, and federal levels. Centering diabetes efforts and interventions on equity will improve diabetes treatment and care for all.

Peer Support to Enhance Type 2 Diabetes Prevention Among African American and Latino Adults 573

Irving Ling, Ruth Enid Zambrana, Sandra Echeverria, and Lenny López

Social support occurs within complex social networks that are diffusely embedded within the social determinants of health. Social networks operate through five primary interconnected pathways: (1) provision of social support; (2) social influence; (3) social engagement; (4) social capital; and (5) social cohesion. Research has demonstrated that increased social support can have a beneficial impact on Type 2 Diabetes (T2DM) prevention and outcomes through culturally tailored Diabetes Prevention Programs in minority communities. Further research is needed to fully measure the impact of social network peer support on T2DM outcomes to better operationalize and scale up community specific interventions.

Interventions Across the Translational Research Spectrum: Addressing Disparities Among Racial and Ethnic Minoritized Youth with Type 1 Diabetes 585

Deborah A. Ellis and Sylvie Naar

Racial and ethnic minoritized youth with type 1 diabetes (T1D) are at elevated risk for health disparities. Few intervention studies have been conducted for these youth and evidence to support best practices to address their needs is lacking. Existing evidence supports the use of brief trials of diabetes technology with structured support from clinic staff, culturally tailored interventions such as language-congruent clinical care, and

use of community health workers as promising directions to improve health outcomes. Clinicians and researchers should work collaboratively with community members to improve the quality of T1D intervention science for racial and ethnic minoritized youth.

Diabetes Care in Humanitarian Settings **603**

Sylvia Kehlenbrink, Kiran Jobanputra, Amulya Reddy, Philippa Boulle, Apoorva Gomber, Rachel Nugent, Vinod Varma, Anna T. Nakayama, and Tom Ellman

Despite the increasing prevalence of diabetes in populations experiencing humanitarian crisis, along with evidence that people living with diabetes are at higher risk for poor outcomes in a crisis, diabetes care is not routinely included in humanitarian health interventions. We here describe 4 factors that have contributed to the inequities and lack of diabetes inclusion in humanitarian programmes: (1) evolving paradigms in humanitarian health care, (2) complexities of diabetes service provision in humanitarian settings, (3) social and cultural challenges, and (4) lack of financing. We also outline opportunities and possible interventions to address these challenges and improve diabetes care among crisis-affected populations.

Equity in Obesity Review **617**

Karla N. Kendrick, Kevin J. Bode Padron, Nichola Z. Bomani, Jashalynn C. German, Dennis D. Nyanyo, Brenda Varriano, Lucy Tu, and Fatima Cody Stanford

Obesity disproportionately affects racial and ethnic minoritized populations and those of lower socioeconomic status. Similarly, disparities exist in the development of its downstream consequences, such as type 2 diabetes and hypertension. The causes of these disparities are multifactorial and are influenced by structural factors such as segregation and healthcare access, and individual-level factors such as weight stigma. Interventions to decrease disparities in obesity should consider macro-level, community, and individual-level factors that might reduce disparities and improve equity in obesity care. Clinicians must also recognize the chronic nature of obesity, and how bias and stigma may impact patient care.

Racial and Ethnic Disparities in Metabolic Bone Disease **629**

Lauren Y. Maldonado, Linette Bosques, Sara J. Cromer, Sharl S. Azar, Elaine W. Yu, and Sherri-Ann M. Burnett-Bowie

Racial and ethnic disparities exist in the prevalence and management of osteoporosis, metastatic cancer, and sickle cell disease. Despite being the most common metabolic bone disease, osteoporosis remains underscreened and undertreated among Black women. Skeletal-related events in metastatic cancer include bone pain, pathologic fractures, and spinal cord compression. Disparities in screening for and treating skeletal-related events disproportionately affect Black patients. Metabolic bone disease contributes significantly to morbidity in sickle cell disease; however, clinical guidelines for screening and treatment do not currently exist. Clinical care recommendations are provided to raise awareness, close health care gaps, and guide future research efforts.

Global Health Disparities in Childhood Rickets 643

Alicia Diaz-Thomas and Pallavi Iyer

Nutritional rickets is a global health problem reflecting both historical and contemporary health disparities arising from racial, ethnic, environmental, and geopolitical circumstances. It primarily affects marginalized populations and can contribute to long-term morbidity. Deficits in bone health in childhood may also contribute to osteomalacia/osteoporosis. Solutions require a global public health approach.

Racial and Ethnic Disparities in Access to and Outcomes of Infertility Treatment and Assisted Reproductive Technology in the United States 659

Gabriela Beroukhim and David B. Seifer

Infertility disproportionately affects the minority, non-White populace, with Black women having twofold higher odds than White women. Despite higher infertility rates, minority racial and ethnic groups access and utilize fertility care less frequently. Even once care is accessed, racial and ethnic disparities exist in infertility treatment and ART outcomes. Preliminary studies indicate that Asian and American Indian women have lower intrauterine insemination pregnancy rates. Many robust studies indicate significant racial and ethnic disparities in rates of clinical pregnancy, live birth, pregnancy loss, and obstetrical complications following in vitro fertilization, with lower favorable outcomes in Black, Asian, and Hispanic women.

Challenges of Gender-Affirming Care in Incarcerated Transgender People 677

Rana Malek, Mauro Sarmiento, and Elizabeth Lamos

Social and health disparities among transgender people may result in increased rates of incarceration, particularly among Black transgender women. The World Professional Association for Transgender Health states that all recommendations for gender-affirming care made in the Standards of Care-8 be applied equally to people living in institutions. Understanding the structural challenges to gender-affirming care in the corrections environment will allow the endocrinologist to navigate the complex correctional health care system. The barriers to gender-affirming care and surgery will be highlighted in this article.

Disparities in Access to High-Volume Surgeons and Specialized Care 689

Terry P. Gao, Rebecca L. Green, and Lindsay E. Kuo

The significant volume–outcome relationship has triggered interest in improving quality of care by directing patients to high-volume centers and surgeons. However, significant disparities exist for different racial/ethnic, geographic, and socioeconomic groups for thyroid, parathyroid, adrenal, and pancreatic neuroendocrine surgical diseases disease.

Sociodemographic Factors in Pituitary Adenomas 705

Adriana G. Ioachimescu

Pituitary adenomas have been increasingly detected in recent years, especially in the older population. Black patients have a higher incidence than other racial groups. In patients with functioning tumors, presentation and

comorbidities are influenced by age and sex, whereas the impact of ethno-racial background is unclear. Active surveillance recommendation and surgery refusal disproportionally affect Black and older patients. The likelihood of surgery at high-volume centers is lower for patients of Black or Hispanic background, uninsured or with lower socioeconomic status. Multicentric studies are necessary to delineate the influence of sociodemographic factors according to the adenoma type and to address the causes of health care disparities.

Hormonal Injustice: Environmental Toxicants as Drivers of Endocrine Health Disparities **719**

Margaret C. Weiss, Luyu Wang, and Robert M. Sargis

The toll of multiple endocrine disorders has increased substantially in recent decades, and marginalized populations bear a disproportionate burden of disease. Because of the significant individual and societal impact of these conditions, it is essential to identify and address all modifiable risk factors contributing to these disparities. Abundant evidence now links endocrine dysfunction with exposure to endocrine-disrupting chemicals (EDCs), with greater exposures to multiple EDCs occurring among vulnerable groups, such as racial/ethnic minorities, those with low incomes, and others with high endocrine disease burdens. Identifying and eliminating EDC exposures is an essential step in achieving endocrine health equity.

ENDOCRINOLOGY AND METABOLISM CLINICS OF NORTH AMERICA

FORTHCOMING ISSUES

March 2024
Type 1 Diabetes
Osagie Ebekozien, *Editor*

June 2024
Early and Late Presentation of Physical Changes of Puberty: Precocious and Delayed Puberty Revisited
Peter Lee and John Fuqua, *Editors*

September 2024
Update on Endocrine Disorders During Pregnancy
Rachel Pessah-Pollack, and
Maria Papaleontiou, *Editors*

RECENT ISSUES

September 2023
Metabolic-Associated Fatty Liver Disease
Sherouk Fouda and Joseph M. Pappachan, *Editors*

June 2023
Endocrinology of the Aging Patient
Rita Rastogi Kalyani, *Editor*

March 2023
Diabetes Remission
Betul Hatipoglu, *Editor*

Foreword
Disparities in Endocrinology Care

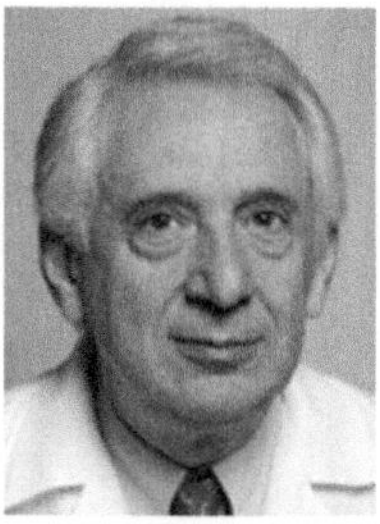

Robert Rapaport, MD
Consulting Editor

Inequities in medicine have been recognized for a very long time. Disparities have received recent attention in all the major journals and even more so in specialty journals. Much has been written about the pandemic's effect and how it highlighted disparities in medical care. This year, it is time to critically examine disparities in endocrinology. At the recently concluded Endocrine Society meeting in Chicago, there was a session devoted to disparities, and a comprehensive article followed. It is therefore time that an issue be devoted to examining health equity in endocrinology. This comprehensive issue devotes, as expected and needed, articles regarding equity in diabetes care from management, peer support for patients with T2 diabetes, disparities in youth with T1 diabetes, and diabetes care in humanitarian settings. In addition, disparities were examined in obesity, in metabolic bone disease, as well as in childhood rickets. Relatively little research has been devoted to less common areas where technology is at the forefront of care. In this issue, advanced reproductive technology for fertility treatment and high-volume surgical procedures is examined. Pituitary adenomas and transgender care are also critically reviewed in this issue. In addition, novel approaches have been included, looking at environmental toxicants and their effects with the prism of health disparities. I

Endocrinol Metab Clin N Am 52 (2023) xiii–xiv
https://doi.org/10.1016/j.ecl.2023.07.004

believe this groundbreaking issue should be of great interest not only to all involved in endocrinology care but also to those working to reduce disparities in medicine.

Robert Rapaport, MD
Professor of Pediatrics
Emma Elizabeth Sullivan Professor of
Pediatric Endocrinology and Diabetes
Icahn School of Medicine at Mount Sinai Director
Emeritus, Division of Pediatric Endocrinology
Diabetes Kravis Children's Hospital at Mount Sinai

E-mail address:
robert.rapaport@mountsinai.org

Preface

Recognizing and Addressing Health Inequities in Endocrinology and Diabetes

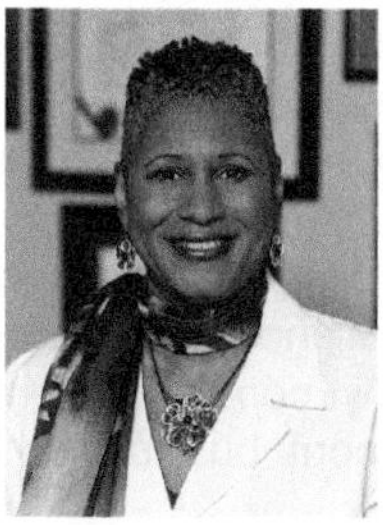
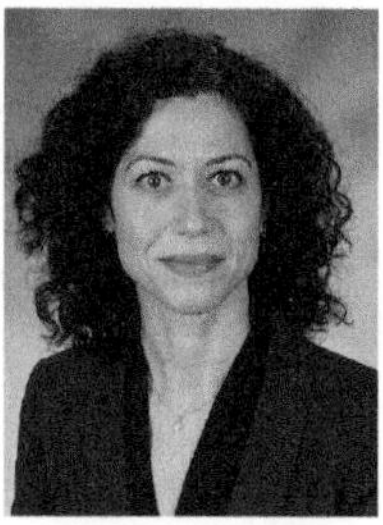

Sherita Hill Golden, MD, MHS   Rana Malek, MD
Editors

In 2020, the American Diabetes Association published a scientific review on Social Determinants of Health (SDOH) and Diabetes,[1] identifying that despite improved treatments, disparities in diabetes care and outcomes persist in minoritized populations. A shift to addressing population health by addressing SDOH has been accelerated by the COVID-19 pandemic. This theme issue of *Endocrinology and Metabolism Clinics of North America* is focused on health equity in endocrinology. In addition to diabetes and obesity, a wider lens to equity in bone disease, reproductive endocrinology, transgender care, endocrine surgery access, and pituitary disease is applied.

Health and health care disparities in diabetes mellitus have been extensively documented, and as summarized by Joseph, these inequities are rooted in SDOH and historical policies that have adversely impacted environmental determinants of diabetes-preventive health behaviors. Therefore, multilevel interventions that target the patient, provider, health system, community, and policy are necessary to achieve health equity for individuals with diabetes. Two articles in this issue describe needed interventions to improve outcomes for minoritized individuals with type 1 and type 2 diabetes. Ling and colleagues describe increasing social support and embedding culturally tailored Diabetes Prevention Program interventions within African American and Latino communities as effective strategies to prevent type 2 diabetes. There are very few intervention studies addressing outcomes in minoritized youth with type 1 diabetes; consequently Ellis and colleagues discuss the need to use community-engaged approaches during intervention development and to ensure that SDOH are addressed as part of the interventions. While more humanitarian crises unfold globally due to climate change and political instability, as well as an increasing prevalence of diabetes within those populations, diabetes care is not routinely included in humanitarian health

Endocrinol Metab Clin N Am 52 (2023) xv–xvii
https://doi.org/10.1016/j.ecl.2023.05.013

interventions. Kehlenbrink and colleagues discuss the challenges faced in delivering diabetes care in humanitarian crisis and opportunities to improve care. Obesity, a primary risk factor for development of type 2 diabetes, disproportionately impacts minoritized individuals, and Kendrick and colleagues point to weight-based bias and stigma as important barriers to care for treatment of obesity that need to be addressed to ensure equitable care.

Addressing global inequities in nutritional rickets are necessary to prevent and delay development of adulthood osteoporosis. Diaz-Thomas indicates that addressing multilevel barriers to adequate calcium and vitamin D are necessary to eradicate rickets globally. Disparities in bone disease persist into adulthood, as described by Maldonado and colleagues, who note underscreening and undertreatment among Black women. The article also highlights a need to address metabolic bone health in sickle cell disease and early management of metastatic bone disease in racial and ethnic minoritized individuals.

Higher rates of infertility exist in racial and ethnic minoritized individuals, who access assisted reproductive technology (ART) at lower rates. Beroukhim and Safer show that even in those women who utilize ART, live birth rates are lower in non-white women, and they identify social, economic, and biologic factors as contributors to those disparities.

Transgender individuals have a high risk for justice system involvement, creating barriers to gender-affirming care when in correctional facilities. Malek and colleagues encourage endocrinologists to understand the structural, interpersonal, and educational barriers to care so that they can support equitable care for transgender individuals who are incarcerated.

Gao and colleagues and Ioachimescu describe disparities in access to high-volume surgeons for endocrine and pituitary disorders. Gao and colleagues note the importance of high-volume surgeons for care given an established volume-outcome relationship for endocrine surgeries. Ioachimescu notes recommendations against surgery and for active surveillance are disproportionately higher for older, Black, Hispanic, and uninsured/underinsured individuals.

The final article by Weiss and colleagues looks broadly at environmental toxicants, in particular, endocrine-disrupting chemicals, and how exposure drives endocrine health disparities. They note that minoritized individuals as well as low-income groups face disproportionate exposure to endocrine disrupting chemicals and describe in detail the various resultant endocrine disorders. The authors also identify tangible recommendations providers can make to reduce exposure to environmental toxins.

Sherita Hill Golden, MD, MHS
Johns Hopkins Medicine
Division of Endocrinology, Diabetes, and Metabolism
Johns Hopkins University School of Medicine
1812 Ashland Avenue, Room 431
Baltimore, MD 21205, USA

Rana Malek, MD
University of Maryland School of Medicine
Division of Endocrinology
Diabetes, and Nutrition
800 Linden Avenue
Baltimore, MD 21201, USA

E-mail addresses:
sahill@jhmi.edu (S.H. Golden)
rmalek@som.umaryland.edu (R. Malek)

REFERENCE

1. Hill-Briggs F, Adler NE, Berkowitz SA, et al. Social determinants of health and diabetes: a scientific review. Diabetes Care 2022;44(1):258–79.

Advancing Equity in Diabetes Prevention, Treatment, and Outcomes

Delivering on Our Values

Joshua J. Joseph, MD, MPH

KEYWORDS

• Diabetes • Health equity • Disparities • Social drivers of health
• Nonmedical health-related social needs

KEY POINTS

- Disparities in diabetes prevention, treatment, and outcomes are rooted in the social drivers of health.
- Advancing diabetes equity requires multimodal interventions addressing multiple levels of the socioecological model.
- All individuals affected by diabetes are needed to advocate for policies to advance diabetes equity.

BACKGROUND

Equitable approaches to health recognize that individuals and communities have varying levels of resources and opportunities for health and allocate the resources needed to achieve equitable outcomes. Thus, equity is based in justice, or the just distribution of resources. Equality-based approaches are defined by equal distribution of resources. Due to the entrenched, enduring, and intersecting challenges of racism, classism, sexism, ableism, cisheteronormativism, urbanism, and other forms of oppression, many individuals and communities have been marginalized, leading to disparities that are difficult to address through equality-based approaches.

Existing disparities are rooted in the Social Drivers (Determinants) of Health (SDoH). SDoH are the conditions in which people are born, grow, live, work, and age. These circumstances are shaped by the distribution of money, power, and resources. SDoH are responsible for greater than 60% to 70% of overall health and have a deleterious influence on health inequities—the unfair and avoidable differences in health.[1,2] Policy is the critical lever to improve SDoH.[3]

Division of Endocrinology, Diabetes and Metabolism, The Ohio State University College of Medicine, Suite 5000E, 700 Ackerman Road, Columbus, OH 43202, USA
E-mail address: Joshua.Joseph@osumc.edu

Endocrinol Metab Clin N Am 52 (2023) 559–572
https://doi.org/10.1016/j.ecl.2023.05.001 endo.theclinics.com

From a diabetes equity lens, ensuring that all people with diabetes have access to quality health care and resources, regardless of race, ethnicity, socioeconomic status, sex, gender, or other protected class characteristics is important. Everyone at risk for or with diabetes should have the opportunity to receive the education, support, treatment, and technology necessary to prevent, manage, and treat diabetes, tailored to their level of need. The process of tailoring the resources requires input from the impacted populations to ensure their solutions are reflected in the strategies. Examples of strategies in marginalized communities include increasing access to affordable health care, healthy food options, and diabetes education and awareness. Few of the existing strategies directly address the root causes of differences, which must be addressed through policy to truly eliminate disparities and advance diabetes equity. Using evidence from the United States (US) non-Hispanic Black (NHB) population as an exemplar, this article will explore the following: (1) disparities in diabetes risk factors, prevention, incidence, prevalence, treatment, and outcomes; (2) root causes of diabetes disparities; and (3) equitable solutions to advance diabetes equity.

DIABETES DISPARITIES

Type 2 diabetes mellitus (diabetes) is characterized by an elevation in blood glucose due to progressive loss of β-cell insulin secretion, on the background of peripheral insulin resistance.[4] Thus, factors that drive insulin resistance are risk factors for diabetes, including adiposity, physical inactivity, poor dietary behaviors, short sleep, smoking, metabolic syndrome components, and family history of diabetes.[4,5] US NHB versus non-Hispanic White (NHW) populations are burdened with more deleterious levels of diabetes risk factors,[6–8] which are encompassed in the American Heart Association (AHA) Life's Essential 8.[9,10]

Even with the disparity in risk factors, the racial/ethnic makeup of the 38% of Americans with prediabetes is proportional to the population,[11] but disparities exist in prevalent diabetes (17.4% NHB and 13.6% NHW).[11] The discordance between prediabetes and diabetes in terms of disparities is driven by a higher incidence of diabetes in NHB populations.[12] In terms of diabetes treatment, only 1 in 5 individuals meet recommended diabetes control targets, including hemoglobin A1c less than 7%, blood pressure less than 140/90 mm Hg and non-HDL cholesterol less than 130 mg/dL. Using the 2023 American Diabetes Association guidelines blood pressure target (<130/80 mm Hg), the percentage is even lower.[13] There are long-standing disparities in glycemic control, with worse control in racial/ethnic minoritized populations.[14,15] The underlying causes for these disparities are hypothesized to be due to differences in socioeconomic, clinical, health care, and self-management factors, along with higher diabetes distress among racial/ethnic minoritized groups but the evidence remains limited and mixed.[14–16]

There has been an explosion in novel medications to treat diabetes during the last 15 to 20 years, including sodium-glucose cotransporter-2 inhibitors, glucagon-like peptide-1 receptor agonists, and selective nonsteroidal mineralocorticoid receptor antagonists, which not only improve glycemia but also lower microvascular and macrovascular risk.[17] Unfortunately, there are significant disparities in prescription of these newer, effective medications among racial/ethnic minoritized and lower socioeconomic status groups, irrespective of insurance status.[18,19] Analyses examining the impact of these disparities on hemoglobin A1c control are an important area of further research.

NHB adults disproportionately develop microvascular complications including retinopathy, nephropathy, and neuropathy.[20] Disparities in chronic kidney disease are particularly concerning, given that a 42% increase in incident cases of end-stage kidney disease occurred between 2000 and 2019 in an era with increasing availability of antihyperglycemic medications that slow glomerular filtration rate decline.[21,22] In regards to cardiovascular disease (CVD), the prevalence of CVD in NHB adults with diabetes is lower than in NHW adults but with similar rates of CVD mortality.[23] Overall, NHB versus NHW Americans have 2-fold higher risk of diabetes mortality, highlighting the importance of CVD and non-CVD mortality in NHB populations.[23]

ROOT CAUSES OF DIABETES DISPARITIES

To address disparities in diabetes by race/ethnicity, socioeconomic status, sex, gender, disability, etc., it is critical to understand and derive solutions focused on root causes, while concurrently addressing systemic and individual factors among individuals and communities made vulnerable by SDoH.[17,24,25] To understand the root causes of present-day inequities in diabetes prevention, treatment, and care, it is paramount to examine the influence of historical factors. For diabetes, we must consider the influences of the past and present sociopolitical context and the mechanisms by which systems and policies have created inequitable opportunities and outcomes.

Of all the "isms" that influence diabetes, racism is one of the leading factors that contribute to diabetes inequities. Many definitions of racism exist but 2 leading scholars in the field define racism in the following ways:

As defined by Dr Camara Jones, "racism is a system of structuring opportunity and assigning value based on the social interpretation of how one looks (which is what we call "race"), that unfairly disadvantages some individuals and communities, unfairly advantages other individuals and communities, and saps the strength of the whole society through the waste of human resources."[26] Dr David Williams notes that structural racism (racial bias among institutions and across society) is the cumulative and compounding effect of an array of societal factors, including the history, culture, ideology, and interactions of institutions and policies that systematically privilege majority populations and disadvantage people of color.[27]

As can be seen from the definitions, there are different contexts or subdefinitions of racism that are important in understanding the intersection with diabetes, including internalized, interpersonal, institutional, and structural racism (**Table 1**). A comprehensive review of the role of various forms of racism in diabetes and endocrinology has been completed[25]; here, we will review the intersection of structural racism, housing, and diabetes as an exemplar.[27]

REDLINING, HOUSING, NEIGHBORHOODS, AND DIABETES

In 1934, the Federal Housing Administration (FHA), through the New Deal's National Housing Act of 1934, promoted homeownership by providing federal backing of loans, which guaranteed mortgages.[28] In 1936, Residential Security Maps were developed by the Home Owners Loan Corporation (HOLC) and adopted by the FHA and Veterans Administration. The maps were color-coded in 4 categories to indicate where it was "safe" to insure mortgages for appraisers.[28] The "Best (A)" neighborhoods were green, "Still Desirable (B)" neighborhoods were blue, "Declining (C)" neighborhoods were yellow, and "Hazardous (D)" neighborhoods were red.[28] The majority of neighborhoods where NHB Americans lived were colored red to indicate to appraisers that these neighborhoods were too risky to insure mortgages and thus, home ownership was denied to millions of NHB Americans. An inextricable link exists between home ownership and wealth because the major asset for most families is their home.[28] Thus, redlining had a major impact on gaps in homeownership and wealth, which persists

Table 1
Definitions of racism

Internalized racism	Racism that lies within individuals based on their private beliefs and biases about race and racism. This involves prejudice toward individuals of a different race, negative beliefs about oneself (internalized oppression) or beliefs about superiority (internalized privilege)
Interpersonal racism	A form of racism that occurs between individuals when their personal racial beliefs affect their public or private interactions. This involves an individual's self-reports of exposure to racist interactions
Institutional racism	A form of racism that occurs within institutions and is mediated through unfair policies and discriminatory practices of institutions resulting in racially inequitable outcomes for racial minority individuals and advantages for white individuals
Structural racism	This refers to racism across institutions and society (at local, state, and federal levels) that is embedded in laws, policies, and practices of society and interactions among its institutions to systematically provide advantage to racial groups deemed as superior while differentially oppressing, disadvantaging racial minority groups

Data from Apollon D, Keheler T, Medeiros J, Lorraine Ortega N, Sebastian J, Sen R. *Moving The Race Conversation Forward: Racial Discourse Change in Practice - Part 2.* Race Forward: The Center for Racial Justice Innovation; 2014. Accessed March 17, 2021. https://act.colorlines.com/acton/attachment/1069/f-0115/1/-/-/-/-/Racial_Discourse_Part_2.PDF.

today. Currently, the homeownership rate is 73% and 42% among NHW and NHB Americans, respectively.[29] NHW families have the highest level of wealth compared with other racial/ethnic groups, while Black families' wealth is less than 15% of NHW families.[30] The far reaching impact of disparities in home ownership and wealth on communities are schools receiving less funding and fewer health promoting businesses (grocery stores, gyms, banks, and so forth; **Fig. 1**). The opportunity to attain health is linked to these social conditions and policies, and the impact is amplified by the additional layer of the medical and scientific contributors to inequities (see **Fig. 1**). In Columbus, Ohio, a large US midwestern metropolitan city, there is a vast overlap between the HOLC map from 1936 and present-day diabetes prevalence and hospital admissions (**Fig. 2**), which is a similar pattern in many US cities. Nationally, there is a graded increase in cardiometabolic disease across HOLC grades (A [green] – D [red]), with redlined neighborhoods having the highest diabetes prevalence, diabetes comorbidities (obesity, hypertension, and smoking), and microvascular and macrovascular outcomes.[31] Further analyses of HOLC and diabetes mortality, showed that (1) a 1-unit higher HOLC grade was associated with a 54% higher diabetes morality rate and 67% higher rate of diabetes years of life lost.[32]

HOLC grades, a historical form of structural racism, may affect diabetes inequities through nonmedical health-related social needs (social needs), defined as the individual social and economic needs such as housing, food, and transportation.[33,34] As described in **Fig. 3**, upstream SDoH factors (structural racism and poverty) influence midstream nonmedical health-related social needs influencing downstream diabetes outcomes. As an example, food and nutrition security are critical in diabetes management, given the impact of dietary macronutrient intake on blood glucose.[35] Food insecurity is a household-level economic and social condition of limited or uncertain access to adequate food.[36] Food insecurity is challenging in diabetes due to negative

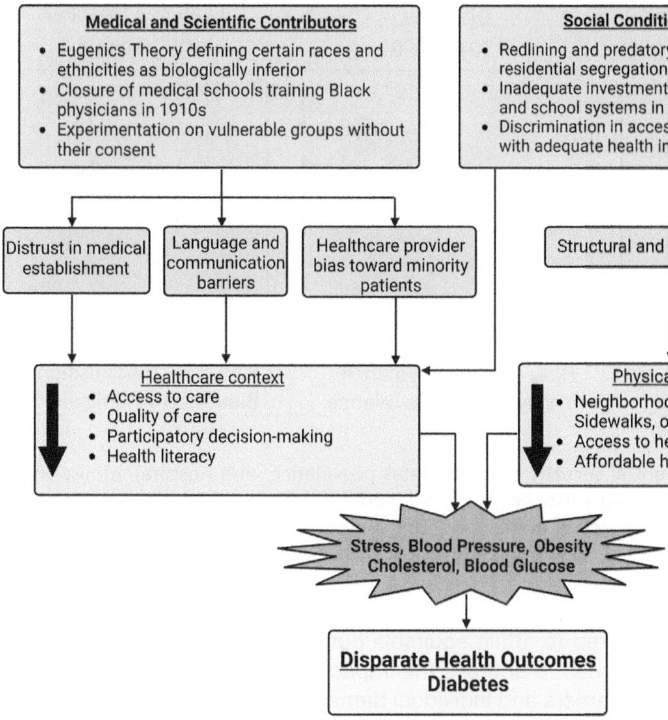

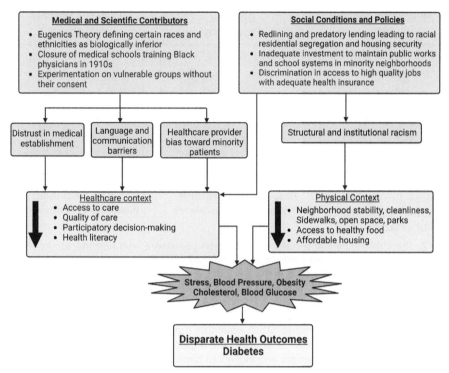

Fig. 1. Medical, scientific, and social policy contributors to health and health-care disparities in African Americans in the United States. Figure shows the medical, scientific, and social policy contributors to health and health-care disparities in African Americans in the United States. (*Adapted from* Golden SH, Joseph JJ, Hill-Briggs F. Casting a Health Equity Lens on Endocrinology and Diabetes. J Clin Endocrinol Metab. 2021;106(4):e1909-e1916; with permission; and *Created with* BioRender.com.)

compensatory eating behaviors (eg, skipping meals, consumption of processed foods, high carbohydrate intake, and poor dietary quality) that instigate periods of hyperglycemia and hypoglycemia; and a resulting increase in risk for poor diabetes self-management.[2,37] The diabetes and food insecurity intersection is unfortunately common with 19% of individuals living with diabetes experiencing food insecurity, with higher rates in lower resourced communities.[2,38] The 1936 HOLC C and D graded areas have over a 2-fold higher odds of food insecurity today.[39] Increases in contemporary census tract proportions of Black, Hispanic, or other racial/ethnic minoritized residents, as well as disabled residents, are associated with reduced food access.[39] Thus, although residential security maps were developed more than 80 years ago, those policy decisions continue to have a devastating impact on diabetes prevalence and outcomes.

SOLUTIONS TO ADVANCING DIABETES EQUITY

"Diabetes equity" ensures that all people at-risk for or with diabetes have access to quality health care and management resources, regardless of underlying sociodemographic factors that drive disparities. Embedded within diabetes equity is the reality that individuals face heterogeneous challenges in preventing and managing diabetes.

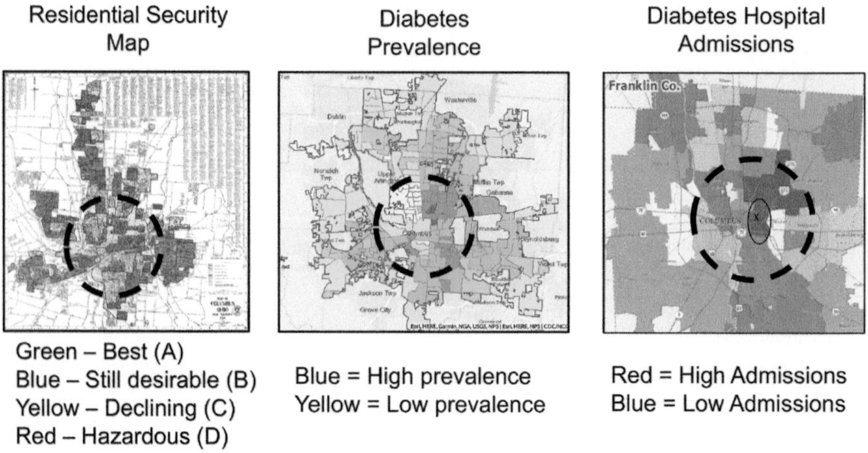

Fig. 2. The 1936 residential security map, diabetes prevalence, and hospital admissions in Columbus, Ohio. An overlap exists between redlined neighborhoods in 1936, present-day diabetes prevalence and hospital admissions. The source for the diabetes prevalence data is the Centers for Disease Control and Prevention 500 Cities Project. (HOLC "redlining" maps. National Archives.)

Thus, the resources required to attain equitable outcomes are going to vary. Many populations require resources to address the impacts of upstream SDoH, including community and societal barriers and individual barriers due to intermediate nonmedical health-related social needs (see **Fig. 3**). Diabetes equity propels us to consider the

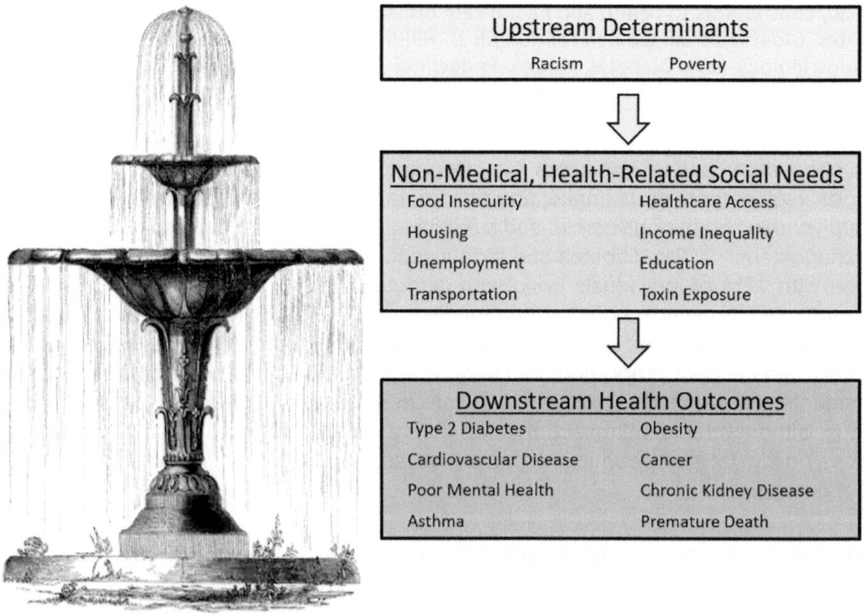

Fig. 3. Upstream determinants, nonmedical health-related social needs, and downstream health outcomes. The figure shows the relationship between upstream determinants, nonmedical health-related social needs, and downstream health outcomes.

individual within the context of their families, friends, organizations, communities, and the broader society, and ultimately to develop multilevel programs and interventions to engage across the socioecological model to advance equity (**Fig. 4**). Thus, solutions should include individual tailoring of education, support, treatment, and technologies to prevent and manage diabetes, along with addressing upstream root causes, including neighborhood environments, structural racism, and poverty, through policy advocacy and change (see **Fig. 4**).

Programs and interventions aimed at improving diabetes equity have included community-based programs, health system interventions, insurance expansion of access to diabetes medication and supplies, public health campaigns (National Diabetes Prevention Program), addressing social needs and policy changes (Affordable Care Act, Inflation Reduction Act).[2,23,40] These interventions have set us on a path to improve diabetes equity but current disparities necessitate continued innovation to eliminating inequities in diabetes incidence, prevalence, treatment, control, and outcomes.

A DIABETES EQUITY EXEMPLAR: BLACK IMPACT

Black men have the shortest life expectancy of any race/sex group, astoundingly 7 years shorter than NHW and Hispanic men,[41,42] and spend a greater number of years living with chronic conditions, including diabetes.[43] CVD is the leading cause of death in Black men and among all individuals with diabetes.[43] Lower attainment of cardiovascular health (CVH), indicated by the AHA Life's Simple 7 (physical activity, diet, cholesterol, blood pressure, body mass index, smoking, and glycemia) and Life's Essential 8 (Life's Simple 7 + sleep),[9,44] is a major contributor to Black men having high diabetes prevalence and the shortest life-expectancy of any race/sex group. In fact, higher attainment of AHA CVH scores has been associated with lower risk of diabetes and diabetes sequelae including CVD, cancer, and mortality.[7,8,45,46] In 2019, a systematic review of community-engaged and community-based participatory research (CBPR) showed that only 2 studies addressed all 7 AHA Life's Simple 7 metrics in Black populations

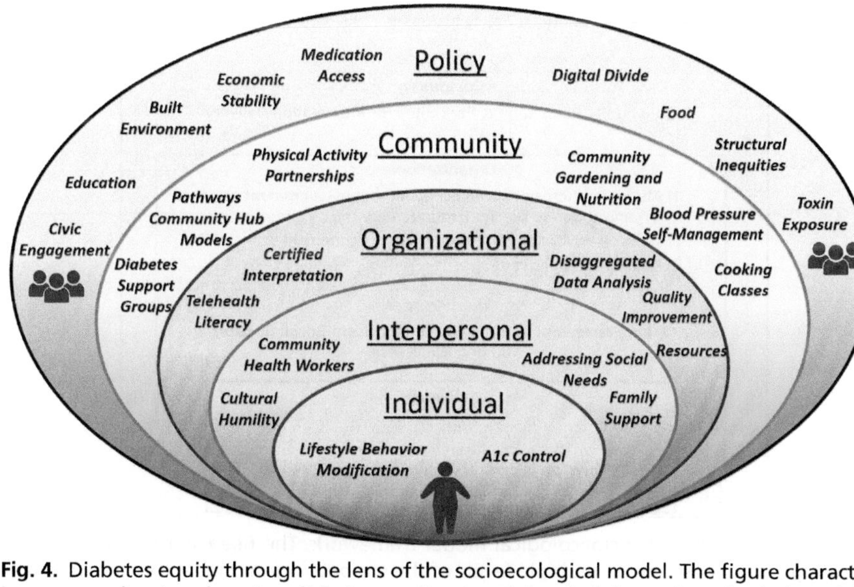

Fig. 4. Diabetes equity through the lens of the socioecological model. The figure characterizes approaches to advancing diabetes equity at each level of the socioecological model.

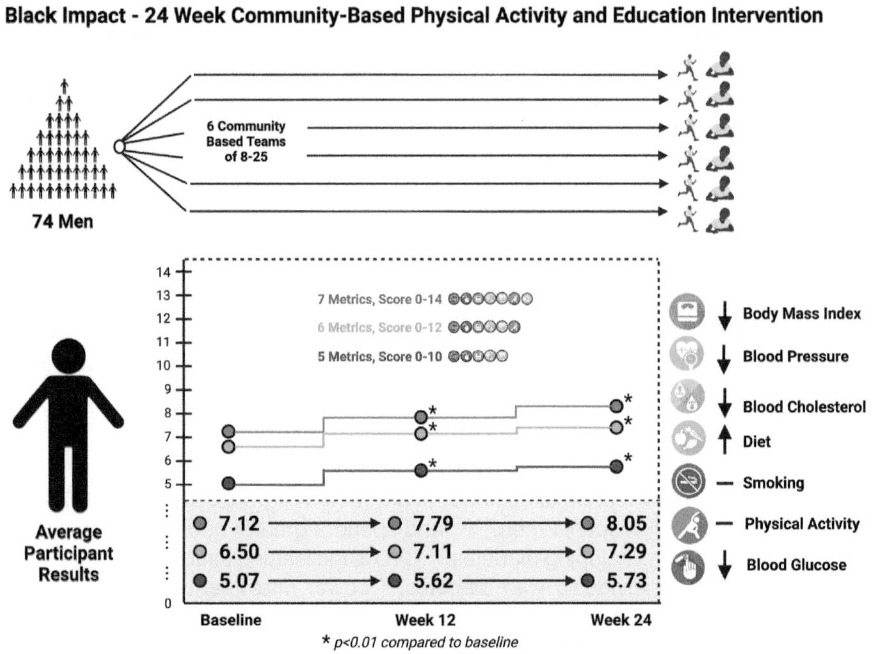

Fig. 5. The Black Impact 24-week community-based intervention. The Black Impact intervention improved multiple measures of cardiometabolic health through physical activity, health education, identifying and addressing social needs, and engaging with primary care. (*Created with* BioRender.com.)

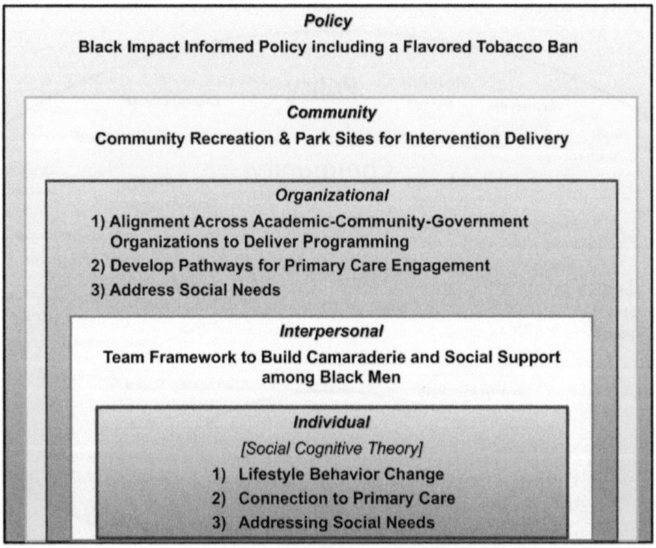

Fig. 6. The Black Impact socioecological model framework. The Black Impact intervention was designed to intervene at multiple levels of the socioecological model to improve cardiometabolic health in Black men.

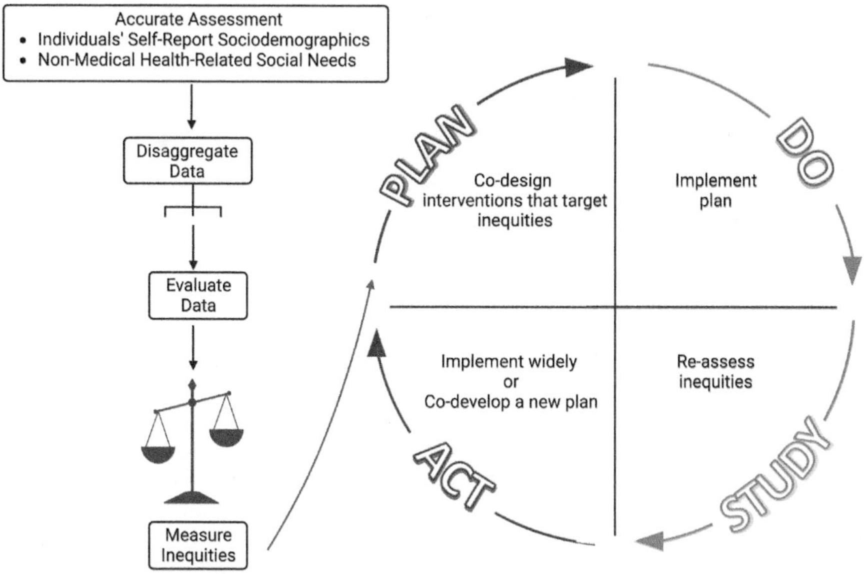

Fig. 7. Strategies to advance diabetes equity through quality improvement and program evaluation. One approach to commence advancing diabetes equity is to accurately assess populations, evaluate disaggregated data for inequities, and then codesign interventions with the population that is impacted by the disparity and proceed through a quality improvement, plan-do-study-act cycle. (*Created with* BioRender.com.)

and neither focused solely on Black men.[47–50] Thus, Academic-Community-Government partners including The African American Male Wellness Agency, Health Impact Ohio, and Columbus Recreation and Parks, among multiple other stakeholders and community members, met to conceive and develop "Black Impact." The Black Impact intervention is adapted from the Diabetes Prevention Program and AHA Check, Change, Control programs based on stakeholder feedback to incorporate additional evidence-based strategies for influencing target outcomes.[51] The 24-week CBPR program focuses on improving attainment of AHA CVH scores in Black men through physical activity, health education, identifying and addressing unmet social needs, and increasing engagement in primary care. Black Impact significantly improved cardiometabolic health including diabetes risk factors such as weight, blood pressure, lipids, and glucose, along with improving dietary intake (**Fig. 5**).[51] Overall, improvements in cardiometabolic health equated to a 19% lower risk of mortality. Additionally, Black Impact reduced social needs, increased patient activation, and leveraged social support.[34,52,53] Black Impact intervened at multiple levels of the socioecological model framework to drive impact and advance health equity in Black men (**Fig. 6**).

SUMMARY

Multilevel, multimodal solutions targeting all levels of the socioecological model framework are equipped to make the largest advances in diabetes equity from a population perspective. Quality improvement and program evaluation studies are also necessary to drive innovation in health care and across populations. Quality improvement and program evaluation studies often begin with disaggregated data analysis identifying disparities in certain populations (**Fig. 7**). Disaggregated data analyses depend on accurate and reliable collection of sociodemographic information. This is a major area of emphasis for the culturally and linguistically appropriate services guidelines in health care.[25,54] Quality improvement proceeds with the development of interventions implemented using the plan-do-study-act method with scaling of successful interventions (see **Fig. 7**). Another pivotal area is advocating for diabetes equity in all organizational, local, state, and federal policies. Policy advocacy requires steadfast engagement of all individuals affected by diabetes from patients to providers to policymakers. Although, big "P" policy decisions such as passage of the Inflation Reduction Act will lead to massive drug savings for older Americans with diabetes,[55] little "p" policy decisions at the organizational and local level such as preferred drug lists are just as important in improving pillars of diabetes equity including pharmacoequity.[56] Policies that improve the neighborhood environment are also germane to diabetes equity and have been shown to improve glycemia.[57] Health-care advocates are pushing to modernize diabetes quality care measures, given that only 1 in 2 individuals is currently meeting targets for glycemia.[58] Redesigning health care, including alternative payment models, value-based arrangements, and diabetes care quality measurement and reporting, would support policies and practices to improve diabetes health overall and diabetes equity.[58,59] Many of these strategies are aligned with the National Clinical Care Commission report to the US Congress in 2023, which adopted a framework that combines elements of the socioecological model with the chronic care model.[60] "The Time is Now" to advance diabetes equity through multilevel, multimodal, cross-disciplinary, partnered, inclusive approaches that center on equity.

CLINICS CARE POINTS

- Screening for and addressing nonmedical health-related social needs is important in advancing diabetes equity.
- Collecting accurate sociodemographic information, disaggregating data and examining outcomes may inform topics for equity-based interventions.
- Health-care providers should stay informed about the impact of federal, state, local, and institutional polices on the treatment, care, and outcomes of individuals with diabetes.

DISCLOSURE

The author has no conflicts of interest to declare.

REFERENCES

1. World Health Organization. World Health Organization: What are the Social Determinants of Health? Available at: https://www.who.int/social_determinants/sdh_definition/en/. Accessed January 3, 2023.
2. Hill-Briggs F, Adler NE, Berkowitz SA, et al. Social determinants of health and diabetes: a scientific review. Diabetes Care 2021;44(1):258–79.
3. Yearby R, Clark B, Figueroa JF. Structural racism in historical and modern US health care policy: study examines structural racism in historical and modern US health care policy. Health Aff 2022;41(2):187–94.
4. ElSayed NA, Aleppo G, Aroda VR, et al. 2. Classification and diagnosis of diabetes: *standards of care in diabetes—2023*. Diabetes Care 2023;46(Supplement_1):S19–40.

5. Joseph JJ, Kluwe B, Echouffo-Tcheugui JB, et al. Association of adiposity with incident diabetes among black adults in the jackson heart study. JAHA 2021; 10(18):e020716.
6. Joseph JJ, Echouffo-Tcheugui JB, Talegawkar SA, et al. Modifiable lifestyle risk factors and incident diabetes in African Americans. Am J Prev Med 2017; 53(5):e165–74.
7. Joseph JJ, Echouffo Tcheugui JB, Carnethon MR, et al. The association of ideal cardiovascular health with incident type 2 diabetes mellitus: the Multi-Ethnic Study of Atherosclerosis. Diabetologia 2016;59(9):1893–903.
8. Joseph JJ, Bennett A, Echouffo Tcheugui JB, et al. Ideal cardiovascular health, glycaemic status and incident type 2 diabetes mellitus: the REasons for Geographic and Racial Differences in Stroke (REGARDS) study. Diabetologia 2019;62(3):426–37.
9. Lloyd-Jones DM, Allen NB, Anderson CAM, et al. Life's Essential 8: updating and enhancing the american heart association's construct of cardiovascular health: a presidential advisory from the American Heart Association. Circulation 2022; 146(5).
10. Lloyd-Jones DM, Ning H, Labarthe D, et al. Status of Cardiovascular Health in US Adults and children using the american heart association's new "life's essential 8" metrics: prevalence estimates from the national health and nutrition examination survey (NHANES), 2013-2018. Circulation 2022;122:060911. https://doi.org/10.1161/CIRCULATIONAHA.122.060911. Published online June 29:CIRCULATIONAHA.
11. Centers for Disease Control and Prevention. National Diabetes Statistics Report 2022. Estimates of Diabetes and Its Burden in the United States. Available at: https://www.cdc.gov/diabetes/data/statistics-report/index.html. Accessed March 8, 2022.
12. Benoit SR, Hora I, Albright AL, et al. New directions in incidence and prevalence of diagnosed diabetes in the USA. BMJ Open Diab Res Care 2019;7(1):e000657.
13. Fang M, Wang D, Coresh J, et al. Trends in diabetes treatment and control in U.S. adults, 1999-2018. N Engl J Med 2021;384(23):2219–28.
14. Smalls BL, Ritchwood TD, Bishu KG, et al. Racial/ethnic differences in glycemic control in older adults with type 2 diabetes: United States 2003–2014. IJERPH 2020;17(3):950.
15. Heisler M. Mechanisms for racial and ethnic disparities in glycemic control in middle-aged and older Americans in the health and retirement study. Arch Intern Med 2007;167(17):1853.
16. Adams AS, Trinacty CM, Zhang F, et al. Medication adherence and racial differences in A1C control. Diabetes Care 2008;31(5):916–21.
17. Joseph JJ, Deedwania P, Acharya T, et al. Comprehensive management of cardiovascular risk factors for adults with type 2 diabetes: a scientific statement from the American heart association. Circulation 2022;145(9):e722–59.
18. Lamprea-Montealegre JA, Madden E, Tummalapalli SL, et al. Association of race and ethnicity with prescription of SGLT2 inhibitors and GLP1 receptor agonists among patients with type 2 diabetes in the veterans health administration system. JAMA 2022;328(9):861.
19. Eberly LA, Yang L, Essien UR, et al. Racial, ethnic, and socioeconomic inequities in glucagon-like peptide-1 receptor agonist use among patients with diabetes in the US. JAMA Health Forum 2021;2(12):e214182.
20. Haw JS, Shah M, Turbow S, et al. Diabetes complications in racial and ethnic minority populations in the USA. Curr Diab Rep 2021;21(1):2.

21. Tuttle KR, Jones CR, Daratha KB, et al. Incidence of chronic kidney disease among adults with diabetes, 2015–2020. N Engl J Med 2022;387(15):1430–1.
22. Ríos Burrows N, Koyama A, Pavkov ME. Reported cases of end-stage kidney disease—United States, 2000–2019. Am J Transplant 2022;22(5):1483–6.
23. Wittwer JA, Golden SH, Joseph JJ. Diabetes and CVD Risk: special considerations in African Americans related to Care. Curr Cardiovasc Risk Rep 2020; 14(10):15.
24. Joseph JJ, Ortiz R, Acharya T, et al. Cardiovascular impact of race and ethnicity in patients with diabetes and obesity. J Am Coll Cardiol 2021;78(24):2471–82.
25. Dhaliwal R, Pereira RI, Diaz-Thomas AM, et al. Eradicating Racism: An Endocrine Society Policy Perspective. J Clin Endocrinol Metab 2022;107(5):1205–15.
26. Jones CP. Toward the Science and practice of anti-racism: launching a national campaign against racism. Ethn Dis 2018;28(Supp 1):231.
27. Apollon D, Keheler T, Medeiros J, et al. *Moving the race conversation forward: racial discourse change in practice - part 2.* race forward. The Center for Racial Justice Innovation; 2014. Available at: https://act.colorlines.com/acton/attachment/1069/f-0115/1/-/-/-/-/Racial_Discourse_Part_2.PDF. Accessed March 17, 2021.
28. Rothstein R. The color of law: a forgotten history of how Our government segregated America. First published as a Liveright paperback 2018. New York, NY, USA: Liveright Publishing Corporation, a Division of W.W. Norton & Company; 2018.
29. Sharkey P, Taylor KY, Serkey Y. The Gaps Between White and Back America, in Charts. The New York Times. Available at: https://www.nytimes.com/interactive/2020/06/19/opinion/politics/opportunity-gaps-race-inequality.html. Published June 19, 2020. Accessed March 13, 2023.
30. Bhutta N, Chang AC, Dettling LJ, et al. Disparities in wealth by race and ethnicity in the 2019 survey of consumer finances. FEDS Notes 2020;2020(2797). https://doi.org/10.17016/2380-7172.2797.
31. Motairek I, Lee EK, Janus S, et al. Historical neighborhood redlining and contemporary cardiometabolic risk. J Am Coll Cardiol 2022;80(2):171–5.
32. Linde S, Walker RJ, Campbell JA, et al. Historic residential redlining and present-day diabetes mortality and years of life lost: the persistence of structural racism. Diabetes Care 2022;45(8):1772–8.
33. National Academies of Sciences, Engineering, and Medicine. 2019. Investing in Interventions That Address Non-Medical, Health-Related Social Needs: Proceedings of a Workshop. Washington, DC: The National Academies Press. https://doi.org/10.17226/25544.
34. Joseph JJ, Gray DM, Williams A, et al. Addressing non-medical health-related social needs through a community-based lifestyle intervention during the COVID-19 pandemic: The Black Impact program. PLoS One 2023;18(3):e0282103. https://doi.org/10.1371/journal.pone.0282103. Campbell JA.
35. Venkatesh KK, Joseph JJ, Clark A, et al. Association of community-level food insecurity and glycemic control among pregnant individuals with pregestational diabetes. Primary Care Diabetes 2023;17(1):73–8.
36. Economic Research Service, United States Department of Agriculture. Definitions of Food Security. Definitions of Food Security. Published May 13, 2021. Available at: https://www.ers.usda.gov/topics/food-nutrition-assistance/food-security-in-the-us/definitions-of-food-security.aspx. Accessed May 12, 2021.
37. Seligman HK, Schillinger D. Hunger and socioeconomic disparities in chronic disease. N Engl J Med 2010;363(1):6–9.

38. Berkowitz SA, Seligman HK, Choudhry NK. Treat or eat: food insecurity, cost-related medication underuse, and unmet needs. Am J Med 2014;127(4): 303–10.e3.
39. Shaker Y, Grineski SE, Collins TW, et al. Redlining, racism and food access in US urban cores. Agric Human Values 2022. https://doi.org/10.1007/s10460-022-10340-3.
40. Joseph JJ, Golden SH. Diabetes in native populations and underserved communities in the USA. In: Dagogo-Jack S, editor. Diabetes mellitus in developing countries and underserved communities. New York, NY, USA: Springer International Publishing; 2017. p. 251–84. Available at: http://link.springer.com/10.1007/978-3-319-41559-8_14. Accessed January 13, 2017.
41. Arias E, Tejada-Vera B, Kochanek K, et al. Provisional life expectancy estimates for 2021. Hyattsville, MD, USA: National Center for Health Statistics (U.S.); 2022. https://doi.org/10.15620/cdc:118999.
42. Arias E, Tejada-Vera B, Ahmad F, et al. Provisional life expectancy estimates for 2020. Hyattsville, MD, USA: Vital Statistics Rapid Release; 2021. https://doi.org/10.15620/cdc:107201. no 15.
43. Virani SS, Alonso A, Aparicio HJ, et al. Heart disease and stroke statistics-2021 update: a report from the american heart association. Circulation 2021;143(8): e254–743.
44. Lloyd-Jones DM, Hong Y, Labarthe D, et al. Defining and setting national goals for cardiovascular health promotion and disease reduction: the american heart association's strategic impact goal through 2020 and beyond. Circulation 2010; 121(4):586–613.
45. Dong C, Rundek T, Wright CB, et al. Ideal cardiovascular health predicts lower risks of myocardial infarction, stroke, and vascular death across whites, blacks, and hispanics: the northern Manhattan study. Circulation 2012;125(24):2975–84.
46. Rasmussen-Torvik LJ, Shay CM, Abramson JG, et al. Ideal Cardiovascular Health Is Inversely Associated With Incident Cancer: The Atherosclerosis Risk in Communities Study. Circulation 2013;127(12):1270–5.
47. Elgazzar R, Nolan TS, Joseph JJ, et al. Community-engaged and community-based participatory research to promote American Heart Association Life's Simple 7 among African American adults: a systematic review. PLoS One 2020;15(9): e0238374.
48. Brewer LC, Balls-Berry JE, Dean P, et al. Fostering African-American Improvement in Total Health (FAITH!): an Application of the American Heart Association's Life's Simple 7™ among Midwestern African-Americans. J Racial Ethn Health Disparities 2017;4(2):269–81.
49. Brewer LC, Hayes SN, Jenkins SM, et al. Improving cardiovascular health among african-americans through mobile health: the FAITH! App Pilot Study. J Gen Intern Med 2019;34(8):1376–8.
50. Brewer LC, Jenkins S, Hayes SN, et al. Community-based, cluster-randomized pilot trial of a cardiovascular mobile health intervention: preliminary findings of the FAITH! trial. Circulation 2022;146(3):175–90.
51. Joseph JJ, Nolan TS, Williams A, et al. Improving cardiovascular health in black men through a 24-week community-based team lifestyle change intervention: the black impact pilot study. Am J Prev Cardiol 2022;9:100315.
52. Addison S, Yang Y, Metlock F, et al. The role of social support in cardiovascular clinical trial participation among black men: black impact. IJERPH 2022;19(19): 12041.

53. Addison S, Williams A, Zhang J, et al. Abstract 9442: increasing patient activation among black american men in a community-based lifestyle intervention pilot: black impact. Circulation 2022;146(Supplement 1):A9442.
54. Golden SH, Joseph JJ, Hill-Briggs F. Casting a health equity lens on endocrinology and diabetes. J Clin Endocrinol Metab 2021;106(4):e1909–16.
55. Narasimmaraj PR, Oseran A, Tale A, et al. Out-of-pocket drug costs for medicare beneficiaries with cardiovascular risk factors/conditions under the inflation reduction Act. J Am Coll Cardiol 2023. https://doi.org/10.1016/j.jacc.2023.02.002. S0735109723002607.
56. Essien UR, Washington DL, Fine MJ. Beyond detecting and understanding disparities in novel diabetes treatment: need for a major shift in pharmacoequity research. JAMA 2022;328(9):836.
57. Ludwig J, Sanbonmatsu L, Gennetian L, et al. Neighborhoods, obesity, and diabetes — a randomized social experiment. N Engl J Med 2011;365(16):1509–19.
58. Jiang DH, O'Connor PJ, Huguet N, et al. Modernizing diabetes care quality measures: analysis examines modernizing diabetes care quality measures. Health Aff 2022;41(7):955–62.
59. Wang S, Weyer G, Duru OK, et al. Can alternative payment models and value-based insurance design alter the course of diabetes in the United States?: Study examines the impact alternative payment models and value-based insurance design may have on Diabetes in America. Health Aff 2022;41(7):980–4.
60. Herman WH, Schillinger D, Bolen S, et al. The national clinical care commission report to congress: recommendations to better leverage federal policies and programs to prevent and control diabetes. Diabetes Care 2023;46(2):255–61.

Peer Support to Enhance Type 2 Diabetes Prevention Among African American and Latino Adults

Irving Ling, MD[a], Ruth Enid Zambrana, PhD[b], Sandra Echeverria, PhD[c], Lenny López, MD, MPH, MDiv[d,*]

KEYWORDS

• Diabetes prevention program • Social networks • Social support • Social cohesion • Social influence • Social capital • Social engagement

KEY POINTS

- Social support occurs within complex social networks which in turn are embedded within and influenced by the social determinants of health.
- Social networks operate through five primary pathways: (1) provision of social support; (2) social influence; (3) social engagement; (4) social capital; and (5) social cohesion.
- Research has demonstrated that increased social support can have a beneficial impact on type 2 diabetes mellitus prevention and outcomes in minoritized groups.
- Culturally tailored Diabetes Prevention Programs that are situated within Latino and African American communities have been demonstrated to help prevent the development of type 2 diabetes.

INTRODUCTION: HEALTH AND HEALTH CARE DISPARITIES AND SOCIAL DETERMINANTS OF HEALTH

In this article, the authors provide an overview of disparities in type 2 diabetes facing Latino and African American communities and explore how social support within social networks can impact type 2 diabetes mellitus (T2DM) prevention and outcomes. Pervasive racial and ethnic disparities in T2DM have been well-documented for decades. As the landmark National Academy of Medicine report, *Unequal Treatment:*

[a] Kaiser Permanente Northern California, 2425 Geary Boulevard, San Francisco, CA 94115, USA; [b] Harriet Tubman Department of Women, Gender and Sexuality Studies, University of Maryland, Consortium on Race, Gender and Ethnicity, Susquehanna Hall, 4200 Lehigh Road Room 4117, College Park, MD 20742, USA; [c] Department of Public Health Education, 437 Coleman Building, 1408 Walker Avenue, Greensboro, NC 27412, USA; [d] University of California San Francisco, San Francisco VA Medical Center, 4150 Clement Street, San Francisco, CA 94121, USA
* Corresponding author. University of California San Francisco, San Francisco VA Medical Center, 4150 Clement Street, San Francisco, CA 94121.
E-mail address: Lenny.lopez@ucsf.edu

Endocrinol Metab Clin N Am 52 (2023) 573–583
https://doi.org/10.1016/j.ecl.2023.05.012
0889-8529/23/Published by Elsevier Inc.

Confronting Racial and Ethnic Disparities in Health Care, published in 2002, there has been a growing empiric evidence based on how racism and the social determinants of health (SDOH) impact health and health care.[1,2] In fact, sociocultural factors are estimated to account for over 50% of health outcomes, whereas clinical care and treatment account for only 10% to 20% of health outcomes.[3]

The National Institute on Minority Health and Health Disparities SDOH model builds on prior biopsychosocial models and incorporates life course in recognition of the long-lasting health effects of socioeconomic exposures (**Fig. 1**). This framework emphasizes the complex multidimensional etiologies of disparities across social ecosystems, highlighting the limitation of individual level focused research and policy. Within this conceptual matrix, social networks, diffusely embedded across communities, can both be influenced by and impact the SDOH.

We examine how social support, as a function of social networks, interplays and synergizes with social capital, social influence, social cohesion, and social engagement to produce changes in health outcomes. Last, we highlight the body of work developed around culturally tailored Diabetes Prevention Programs (DPPs) for Latino and African American communities to demonstrate how social network theory can be operationalized to reduce health disparities by addressing opportunities and challenges across SDOH.

DISPARITIES IN TYPE 2 DIABETES MELLITUS FOR LATINO AND AFRICAN AMERICAN COMMUNITIES

In the United States, 37.3 million people have diabetes (11.3% of the population) and 96 million adults have prediabetes (38.0% of the adult population). An estimated

National Institute on Minority Health and Health Disparities Research Framework

		Levels of Influence[a]			
		Individual	Interpersonal	Community	Societal
Domains of Influence (Over the Lifecourse)	Biological	Biological Vulnerability and Mechanisms	Caregiver–Child Interaction Family Microbiome	Community Illness Exposure Herd Immunity	Sanitation Immunization Pathogen Exposure
	Behavioral	Health Behaviors Coping Strategies	Family Functioning School/Work Functioning	Community Functioning	Policies and Laws
	Physical/Built Environment	Personal Environment	Household Environment School/Work Environment	Community Environment Community Resources	Societal Structure
	Sociocultural Environment	Sociodemographics Limited English Cultural Identity Response to Discrimination	Social Networks Family/Peer Norms Interpersonal Discrimination	Community Norms Local Structural Discrimination	Social Norms Societal Structural Discrimination
	Health Care System	Insurance Coverage Health Literacy Treatment Preferences	Patient–Clinician Relationship Medical Decision-Making	Availability of Services Safety Net Services	Quality of Care Health Care Policies
Health Outcomes		Individual Health	Family/ Organizational Health	Community Health	Population Health

Fig. 1. National Institute on Minority Health and Health Disparities (NIMHD) social determinants research framework. [a]Health Disparity Populations: Race. Ethnicity, Low SES, Rural, Sexual and Gender Minority. Other Fundamental Characteristics: Sex and Gender, Disability, Geographic Region. (*From* National Institute on Minority Health and Health Disparities. NIMHD Research Framework. December 8, 2022. Accessed December 8, 2022. https://nimhd.nih.gov/researchFramework.)

14.6 million Latinos and 12.4 million African Americans have prediabetes, which is nearly a quarter of their respective US populations.[4] Across adult non-White men and women, the age-adjusted prevalence of diagnosed diabetes was second highest in African Americans (12.1%) and third highest in Latino populations (11.8%).[5] Compared with White adults, Latinos are twice as likely to have T2DM (17% vs 8%).[5] Significant heterogeneity of class, race, and national origin exists within the US Latino population, with a higher prevalence of diabetes among Mexicans (14.4%) and Puerto Ricans (12.4%), whereas Central and South Americans and Cubans had a lower prevalence of 8.3% and 6.5%, respectively.[5]

Large racial disparities exist among African Americans and Latinos across multiple T2DM risk factors, such as obesity, with nearly 50% of Black adults having obesity compared with 42.2% of White adults.[6] Latino women are 20% more likely to be overweight compared with White women.[7] Studies show that although African Americans had higher hypertension prevalence and similar rates of treatment to Whites, they had 30% less blood pressure control; although Latinos had similar prevalence of hypertension compared with Whites, they experienced roughly 20% to 30% less awareness, treatment, and control of their hypertension compared with Whites.[8] Moreover, African Americans have a substantially higher risk of diabetes-related complications such as end-stage renal disease and amputations.[6] In the aftermath of the COVID-19 pandemic, Latinos experienced an increase of 67.5% in excess diabetes-related mortality from 2020 to 2021, which was nearly three times that of Whites, and African Americans experienced an increase of excess diabetes mortality more than twice that of Whites.[9] In light of these disparities occurring across SDOH, it is important to examine how social networks and support can be leveraged to improve health equity for African American and Latino communities.

SOCIAL NETWORKS AND SOCIAL SUPPORT: DEFINITIONS AND MECHANISMS OF ACTION

Social networks are the web of social relationships that surround an individual and are defined by the structure of ties that connect individuals to each other. These ties can be characterized, for example, by the frequency of contact, type of contact, reciprocity of ties, duration, multiplexity (the number of types of transactions or support flowing through a set of ties), and bridging (existence of a path between a node in one group and a node in another group). In turn, networks, as a whole, have characteristics such as size, density (the number of ties between network members divided by the number of possible ties), homogeneity, structural cohesion (number of independent paths that hold together group members), and clustering and segregation (presence of groups within networks).[10] Social networks are also patterned by race/ethnicity. National survey data have shown that White adults have social networks of greater size, diversity, and socioeconomic status and wealth compared with Latinos and African Americans.[11]

The concept that resources embedded in social networks may affect health is drawn from the Social Network Theory of Capital, which posits that individuals benefit from values and social resources that a network fosters.[12] Social networks operate through five primary pathways: (1) provision of social support; (2) social influence; (3) social engagement; (4) social capital (access to information, resources, and material goods); and (5) social cohesion.[13] These pathways in turn impact health by influencing direct physiologic stress responses, health-promoting (ie, healthy diet, health service utilization) and health-damaging behaviors (ie, tobacco use, no exercise), and psychological mechanisms (ie, self-efficacy, self-esteem, coping, depression, and emotional regulation).

As **Fig. 2** highlights, social networks are embedded within larger historic, social, and cultural contexts, in which the SDOH operate. However, networks are modified by the SDOH in ways not often addressed nor analyzed in social support interventions for T2DM. This finding is important because systematic reviews and meta-analyses of clinical trials of social network interventions in T2DM report that group-based initiatives largely use single-person behavior change theories, such as self-efficacy and self-regulation.[14] Yet, the primary analytic lens in these studies is deployed without the inclusion of broader network characteristics in relation to their impacts on health outcomes. For example, adverse neighborhood conditions may favor isolation rather than social support or that individuals living in neighborhoods where people are more likely to help their neighbors are also more likely to receive preventive services.[15] Furthermore, few interventions use all mechanisms of social network support identified above or consider the multilevel embeddedness of social networks in unique social contexts.[16] The complexity of network embeddedness and the incomplete measurement of these factors may partially explain why some studies of social support and health may have modest, null, or conflicting findings. In addition, networks

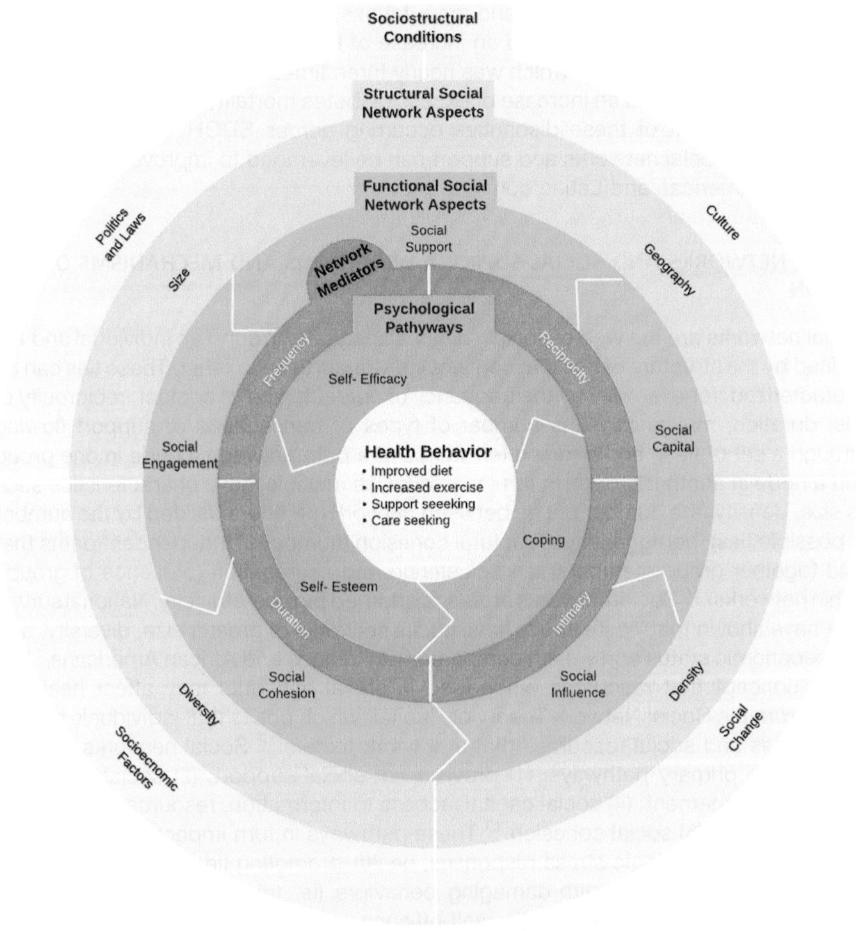

Fig. 2. Model of social network–SDOH interactions for health behaviors.

embody complex, multilevel social interactions between individuals and institutions and may have "emergent properties" not explained by the constituent parts, thus contributing additional confounding to study results.[17]

Social support measures distinguish between the perception of what support is available, the adequacy of potential support, and the extent to which support is received. Social support is further divided into subtypes that include emotional, instrumental, appraisal, and informational support.[18] Emotional support is related to the affective dimensions of love/caring, sympathy, and understanding that close relationships provide. Instrumental support refers to assistance with tangible needs such as transportation to appointments. Appraisal support refers to help in decision-making and giving appropriate feedback as needed. Informational support is related to the provision of advice for self-management decision making. Although some of these types of social support may be difficult to disaggregate, they are useful categories in conceptualizing how support is tangibly provided both cognitively and behaviorally.[18] Higher levels of perceived social support are associated with effective diabetes self-management and increased self-efficacy of self-management behaviors, better glycemic control, and improved quality of life.[19,20] The lack of social support is associated with increased mortality and diabetes-related complications.[21]

Many programs and interventions that seek to prevent diabetes or improve diabetes self-management in the community setting build on providing social support and draw on four closely related social concepts: social capital, social cohesion, social influence, and social engagement. Social capital is defined as the features of social structures that serve as resources for collective action (eg, interpersonal trust, reciprocity norms, and mutual aid).[22] Research shows that lower socioeconomic status individuals tend to use local, strong, and family ties that in turn reinforce poor social capital. Social cohesion refers to the extent of connectedness and solidarity among groups in a community. In the African American Jackson Heart Study, higher neighborhood social cohesion was associated with a 22% lower incidence of T2DM.[23] Social influence refers to the process of interpersonal influence between actors due to normative attitudes and behaviors embedded in the social context. Shared norms around health behaviors, such as, dietary patterns, might be strong sources of social influence. For example, in the Framingham Heart Study, a person's chances of becoming obese increased by 57% if a friend also became obese in a given interval.[24] Interventions that are community-based, such as faith-based organizations (FBOs), can also increase social engagement, which contributes overall to instrumental and informational social support, such as food pantries or informational sessions held at churches.

Family and partners play an important role in the management of diabetes. Those with higher marital satisfaction reported higher diabetes-related satisfaction and felt that diabetes had less of a negative impact on their lives.[25] One study of African Americans found that family belief in an optimistic worldview and sense of togetherness has a positive effect on diabetes self-management and greater physical activity, higher morale including fewer depressive symptoms, higher self-assessed general health, and better quality of life.[26] Family structure and traditions were associated with healthy eating and exercise among Latinos with diabetes.[27] However, tension and stress in family and partner relationships can hinder engagement in self-management behaviors, such as nonsupport for dietary changes, emotional distress, and the creation of increased role demands in caregiving.[28,29] Persons with diabetes may experience family members without diabetes as overprotective or unsupportive.[30]

Other peers can also provide social support for diabetes self-management. Peer support has been broadly defined as "support from a person who has experiential knowledge of a specific behavior or stressor and similar characteristics as the target population."[31] Examples of shared characteristics include age, gender, disease status, socioeconomic status, religion, and ethnicity. This shared background facilitates social support through the exploration of feelings, problem-solving, goal setting, self-efficacy, and hence self-management success through more horizontal power dynamics.

Community health workers (CHWs) are frontline trained public health workers who serve as peer support bridges between their ethnic, cultural, or geographic communities and health care providers and engage their community to prevent and treat diabetes and its complications through education, lifestyle changes, self-management behaviors, and social support. The use of CHWs and their many variants (ie, peer counselors or *promotoras*) has been shown to improve diabetes outcomes in Latino and African American populations.[32] For example, the DIALBEST trial used CHWs to deliver 17 individual sessions on healthy lifestyle and demonstrated improvements in A1C sustained through 6 month post-intervention follow-up.[33]

DIABETES PREVENTION PROGRAM INTERVENTIONS BUILDING ON SOCIAL SUPPORT

A primary national example of peer support-based social network interventions for the prevention of T2DM has been the National DPP. The 2002 US DPP study demonstrated that modest lifestyle changes, including participation in at least 150 minutes of activity per week, resulted in greater than 7% weight loss and significantly reduced the progression of prediabetes to diabetes.[34] In March 2010, Congress authorized the Centers for Disease Control and Prevention (CDC) to create the national DPP to offer evidenced-based, cost–effective, and community-based interventions across the country to prevent T2DM.[35] This program targeted adults who had prediabetes, gestational diabetes, or had other high-risk factors for the development of T2DM. The national DPP runs as a 1-year program with weekly to biweekly sessions that include three key components: (1) CDC-approved curriculum around health and nutrition, (2) a lifestyle coach who is trained to lead the program, and (3) a support group of peers with similar goals and challenges.[36] Ten-year follow-up findings from the initial DPP cohort demonstrated that DPP participants continued to have a delay of development of diabetes by 34% and developed diabetes 4 years later compared with those in the control arm. For participants ages 60 years and older, there was a delay in development by 49%.[37] Although the DPP still continues to serve as a central framework for diabetes prevention, racial and ethnic disparities in program efficacy exist, as African American participants were less likely to meet the 5% weight loss goal (odds ratio [OR] 0.489, $P < .0001$) and Latino participants were less likely to meet the 150 minute per week activity goal (OR 0.952, $P < .0001$) compared with White participants.[38]

In the last decade, there have been several pilot studies and randomized controlled trials that explore the role of culturally appropriate adaptations of the DPP through cultural targeting and tailoring. Some studies involve translating English language materials and providing sessions in participant's native languages where others involve community-based participation in redesigning and adapting DPP to the community. Reviews of culturally tailored DPPs among African American and Latino communities report that most of the programs are moderately effective in reducing A1C, weight, and body mass index. One review identified that successful programs were able to tailor interventions across four major domains of facilitators, location, language, and messaging, whereas less successful programs only tailored interventions across a limited number of these domains.[39] Furthermore, multiple reviews also highlighted the importance of CHWs as facilitators within programs targeting low-income and African American and Latino communities as CHWs could improve the participants' relationship to the program by synergizing efforts across language, location, and messaging. Particularly in DPPs focused on Latino populations, CHWs were present in most studies and could provide literacy-adjusted curriculum, address cultural beliefs regarding diabetes, and leverage friend/family participation within a larger framework of language and cultural concordance that included translation of materials and adapting dietary education to be inclusive of ethnic foods.[39,40] Across studies, there was a wide array of how frequently and deeply CHWs interacted with participants as limited by factors, such as funding and hours, and it was noted that in some studies with less program success, there was less CHW interface.[40]

Culturally important program locations are central to programming in the majority of studies and are important to the success of targeted programs vis-à-vis convenience, familiarity, and safety.[39] Collaborations with FBOs, such as churches, are a central component in DPPs tailored to African Americans.[6] Historically, FBOs have served as integral community nexuses for racial solidarity and civic activity for African Americans. Among African Americans who attend religious services, 60% practice with African American congregations, in which most attendees and senior religious leaders are African American.[41] Data also suggest that African Americans are more religious than the general American public and more likely to credit African American Christian and Muslim organizations as having important roles for advancing the equity of African Americans in the United States.[41]

In addition to these factors, preexisting social networks of FBOs can also aid in DPP goals of modifying health behaviors. In a systematic review of obesity reduction programs targeting African Americans, almost two-thirds of faith-based (incorporation of religious practice and belief within interventions) and faith-placed (secular interventions taking place within the FBO) programming reported statistically significant reductions in weight.[42] Although there were programs that operated from individual to congregation levels, results did not show that multilevel approaches generated greater impact than single-level approaches. Evidence suggests that both individual and group-based interventions within FBO collaborations could be effective for lifestyle change.[42] The structure of FBOs may also serve as a strength for culturally tailored DPPs for African Americans. A pilot study of 352 participants within an African American church reported that exposure to religiously tailored materials and pastoral sermons on diabetes were significantly associated with the greatest overall weight loss among participants.[43]

Overall, culturally tailored DPPs have been shown to be effective with small to moderate effect sizes, which in the context of cardiometabolic risk reduction can have potential clinically meaningful improvement in health.[40] However, the main limitation of peer support interventions has been the considerable heterogeneity in program structure, including contact approach (ie, in-person, via telephone, via email), frequency, duration, degree of intervention strictness (ie, structured vs semi-structured curriculum), and the interventional content provided (ie, information, emotional and appraisal support).[44] There is also no systematic gold standard by which culturally tailored program performance can be measured against. This variability in study design has contributed to the modest findings in systematic reviews and meta-analyses for peer support and diabetes self-management and outcomes. Because targeted peer support and CHW interventions are inherently contextually specific to factors, such as location, culture, and language, it will be important to address the gaps in the literature regarding what programmatic domains may have greater impact across various populations, that is, language may be more integral to Latino participants compared with African American participants.[40]

Furthermore, there is a dearth of studies that measure the degree of impact that DPP interventions have on individuals' social capital, cohesion, and influence as they shape health behaviors leading to improved health outcomes. Although culturally tailored DPP interventions are informed by the theory of social networks, more interdisciplinary approaches will be needed to distill the impacts of DPP models of care within broader social contexts and not just health outcomes alone. Being able to better identify these social nodes and the relational valences between people, places, and spaces will further optimize the operationalization of social network theory in advancing DPP program design and scalability. Future studies should use multisite and multilevel approaches to increase generalizability and adaptability of peer social support interventions beyond general principles.

SUMMARY

This review highlights the importance of the breadth and complexity of how social support is formed and embedded across social networks spanning entire ecosystems as well as how these ecological contexts are shaped by systems to produce inequity. Although numerous disparities in T2DM and metabolic risk factors remain for Latino and African American communities, there are exciting and growing bodies of research looking at how social connections can be used to promote health equity. Ultimately, social support and social networks and their relation to SDOH can have considerable effects on health outcomes in marginalized communities, particularly in regard to the prevention of T2DM. However, further interdisciplinary work, attuned to SDOH, social network analysis, and health outcomes across the intersections of geography, race, ethnicity, and socioeconomic status, are needed to bridge the gaps in our understanding. Social support will also continue to be an important and generative area for health policy as more health care systems recognize the importance of funding and leveraging social networks interventions to promote health through innovations, such as incentivized CHW benefits and adoption of telehealth tools.

CLINICS CARE POINT

- Clinical providers should assess patient's level of social support and engage members of the patients' social network in their type 2 diabetes (T2DM) management and refer their patients at risk for T2DM to culturally tailored Diabetes Prevention Programs if available.

CONFLICT OF INTEREST

The authors have no conflicts of interest to disclose.

REFERENCES

1. Institute of Medicine (US). In: Smedley BD, Stith AY, Nelson AR, editors. Committee on understanding and eliminating racial and ethnic disparities in health care. *Unequal treatment: confronting Racial and ethnic Disparities in health care*. National Academies Press (US); 2003. Available at: http://www.ncbi.nlm.nih.gov/books/NBK220358/. Accessed March 7, 2023.
2. Zambrana RE, Williams DR. The Intellectual Roots Of Current Knowledge On Racism And Health: Relevance To Policy And The National Equity Discourse. Health Aff 2022;41(2):163–70. https://doi.org/10.1377/hlthaff.2021.01439.
3. Marmot M, Allen JJ. Social Determinants of Health Equity. Am J Public Health 2014;104(Suppl 4):S517–9. https://doi.org/10.2105/AJPH.2014.302200.

4. National Diabetes Statistics Report. Estimates of diabetes and its burden in the United States 2020. Published online 2020.
5. Prevalence of Diagnosed Diabetes | Diabetes | CDC. Published September 21, 2022. Available at: https://www.cdc.gov/diabetes/data/statistics-report/diagnosed-diabetes.html. Accessed March 7, 2023.
6. Williams LB, Moser DK, Gustafson A, et al. Reaching high-risk Black adults for diabetes prevention programming during a pandemic: The design of Fit & Faithful a randomized controlled community trial. Contemp Clin Trials 2022;123:106973.
7. Obesity and Hispanic Americans - The Office of Minority Health. Available at: https://minorityhealth.hhs.gov/omh/browse.aspx?lvl=4&lvlid=70. Accessed March 7, 2023.
8. Aggarwal R, Chiu N, Wadhera RK, et al. Racial/Ethnic Disparities in Hypertension Prevalence, Awareness, Treatment, and Control in the United States, 2013 to 2018. Hypertension 2021;78(6):1719–26.
9. Lv F, Gao X, Huang AH, et al. Excess diabetes mellitus-related deaths during the COVID-19 pandemic in the United States. eClinicalMedicine 2022;54. https://doi.org/10.1016/j.eclinm.2022.101671.
10. Prell C. Social network analysis. SAGE Publications, Inc.; 2011. Available at: https://uk.sagepub.com/en-gb/eur/social-network-analysis/book231856. Accessed March 7, 2023.
11. Child ST, Albert MA. Social Networks and Health Outcomes: Importance for racial and socioeconomic disparities in cardiovascular outcomes. Curr Cardiovasc Risk Rep 2018;12(12):30.
12. Lin N, Lin N. Inequality in Social Capital. In; 2017. https://www.semanticscholar.org/paper/Inequality-in-Social-Capital-Lin-Lin/eefe78282f4ae9ad7c31cc39df28cf02969844d1. Accessed March 7, 2023.
13. Berkman LF, Krishna A. Social Network Epidemiology. In: Berkman LF, Kawachi I, Glymour MM, editors. Social epidemiology. Oxford University Press; 2014. p. 0. https://doi.org/10.1093/med/9780195377903.003.0007.
14. Foss C, Knutsen I, Kennedy A, et al. Connectivity, contest and the ties of self-management support for type 2 diabetes: a meta-synthesis of qualitative literature. Health Soc Care Community 2016;24(6):672–86.
15. Prentice JC. Neighborhood effects on primary care access in Los Angeles. Soc Sci Med 2006;62(5):1291–303.
16. Spencer-Bonilla G, Ponce OJ, Rodriguez-Gutierrez R, et al. A systematic review and meta-analysis of trials of social network interventions in type 2 diabetes. BMJ Open 2017;7(8):e016506.
17. Smith KP, Christakis NA. Social Networks and Health. Annu Rev Sociol 2008;34(1):405–29.
18. Lakey B, Cohen S. Social Support Theory and Measurement. In: Cohen S, Underwood LG, Gottlieb BH, editors. Social support measurement and intervention: a guide for health and social scientists, 0. Oxford University Press; 2000. https://doi.org/10.1093/med:psych/9780195126709.003.0002.
19. Soto SC, Louie SY, Cherrington AL, et al. An ecological perspective on diabetes self-care support, self-management behaviors, and hemoglobin A1C among Latinos. Diabetes Educ 2015;41(2):214–23.
20. Strom JL, Egede LE. The impact of social support on outcomes in adult patients with type 2 diabetes: a systematic review. Curr Diab Rep 2012;12(6):769–81.
21. Ciechanowski P, Russo J, Katon WJ, et al. Relationship Styles and Mortality in Patients With Diabetes. Diabetes Care 2009;33(3):539–44.

22. Berkman Lisa F, Kawachi Ichiro, Maria Glymour M, editors. Social epidemiology. 2nd edition. Oxford Academic; 2014.
23. Gebreab SY, Hickson DA, Sims M, et al. Neighborhood social and physical environments and type 2 diabetes mellitus in African Americans: The Jackson Heart Study. Health Place 2017;43:128–37.
24. Christakis NA, Fowler JH. The spread of obesity in a large social network over 32 years. N Engl J Med 2007;357(4):370–9.
25. Trief PM, Wade MJ, Britton KD, et al. A prospective analysis of marital relationship factors and quality of life in diabetes. Diabetes Care 2002;25(7):1154–8.
26. Chesla CA, Fisher L, Mullan JT, et al. Family and disease management in African-American patients with type 2 diabetes. Diabetes Care 2004;27(12):2850–5.
27. Fisher L, Chesla CA, Skaff MM, et al. The family and disease management in Hispanic and European-American patients with type 2 diabetes. Diabetes Care 2000;23(3):267–72.
28. Paddison C. Family support and conflict among adults with type 2 diabetes. Eur Diabetes Nurs 2010;7(1):29–33.
29. Maillet NA, D'Eramo Melkus G, Spollett G. Using focus groups to characterize the health beliefs and practices of black women with non-insulin-dependent diabetes. Diabetes Educ 1996;22(1):39–46.
30. de Ridder DTD, Schreurs KMG, Kuijer RG. Is spousal support always helpful to patients with asthma or diabetes? A prospective study. Psychol Health 2005; 20(4):497–508.
31. Dennis CL. Peer support within a health care context: a concept analysis. Int J Nurs Stud 2003;40(3):321–32.
32. Palmas W, March D, Darakjy S, et al. Community Health Worker Interventions to Improve Glycemic Control in People with Diabetes: A Systematic Review and Meta-Analysis. J Gen Intern Med 2015;30(7):1004–12.
33. Pérez-Escamilla R, Damio G, Chhabra J, et al. Impact of a community health workers-led structured program on blood glucose control among Latinos with type 2 diabetes: The DIALBEST Trial. Diabetes Care 2015;38(2):197–205.
34. Knowler WC, Barrett-Connor E, Fowler SE, et al. Reduction in the incidence of type 2 diabetes with lifestyle intervention or metformin. N Engl J Med 2002; 346(6):393–403.
35. Key National DPP Milestones | National Diabetes Prevention Program | Diabetes | CDC. Published December 27, 2022, Available at: https://www.cdc.gov/diabetes/prevention/milestones.htm. Accessed March 7, 2023.
36. CDC. Lifestyle change program details. Centers for Disease Control and Prevention; 2022. Available at: https://www.cdc.gov/diabetes/prevention/lcp-details.html. Accessed March 7, 2023.
37. Diabetes Prevention Program (DPP) - NIDDK. National Institute of Diabetes and Digestive and Kidney Diseases. Available at: https://www.niddk.nih.gov/about-niddk/research-areas/diabetes/diabetes-prevention-program-dpp. Accessed March 7, 2023.
38. Ely EK, Gruss SM, Luman ET, et al. A National Effort to Prevent Type 2 Diabetes: Participant-Level Evaluation of CDC's National Diabetes Prevention Program. Diabetes Care 2017;40(10):1331–41.
39. Lagisetty PA, Priyadarshini S, Terrell S, et al. Culturally Targeted Strategies for Diabetes Prevention in Minority Population. Diabetes Educ 2017;43(1):54–77.
40. McCurley JL, Gutierrez AP, Gallo LC. Diabetes Prevention in U.S. Hispanic Adults: A Systematic Review of Culturally Tailored Interventions. Am J Prev Med 2017;52(4): 519–29.

41. Mitchell T. Faith Among Black Americans. Pew Research Center's Religion & Public Life Project. Published February 16, 2021. Available at: https://www.pewresearch.org/religion/2021/02/16/faith-among-black-americans/. Accessed March 7, 2023.
42. Lancaster KJ, Carter-Edwards L, Grilo S, et al. Obesity interventions in African American faith-based organizations: a systematic review: Faith-based obesity programmes in blacks. Obes Rev 2014;15:159–76.
43. Berkley-Patton J, Bowe Thompson C, Bauer AG, et al. A Multilevel Diabetes and CVD Risk Reduction Intervention in African American Churches: Project Faith Influencing Transformation (FIT) Feasibility and Outcomes. J Racial Ethn Health Disparities 2020;7(6):1160–71.
44. Dale JR, Williams SM, Bowyer V. What is the effect of peer support on diabetes outcomes in adults? A systematic review. Diabet Med J Br Diabet Assoc 2012;29(11):1361–77.

Interventions Across the Translational Research Spectrum

Addressing Disparities Among Racial and Ethnic Minoritized Youth with Type 1 Diabetes

Deborah A. Ellis, PhD[a,*], Sylvie Naar, PhD[b]

KEYWORDS

• Type 1 diabetes • Youth • Racial and ethnic minorities • Translational research

KEY POINTS

- Insufficient numbers of intervention studies focusing on racial and ethnic minoritized youth with type 1 diabetes (T1D) have been conducted across all stages of translational research.
- Efforts to develop effective interventions for this population should use community-engaged research strategies during early intervention development and include intervention content that addresses social determinants of health.
- New models that do not rely on traditional, phased approaches may be needed to accelerate the pace of developing and disseminating efficacious interventions for racial and ethnic minoritized youth with T1D.

INTRODUCTION

Type 1 diabetes (T1D) is one of the most common chronic illnesses of childhood.[1] The incidence of pediatric T1D has increased in recent years,[2] and the rate of diagnosis among racial and ethnic minoritized youth is increasing at a faster rate than that found in White children.[3] Racial and ethnic minoritized youth with T1D are at elevated risk for health disparities, including suboptimal glycemic control.[4,5] The purpose of this article is to provide a comprehensive review of current interventions to improve the diabetes health of racial and ethnic minoritized youth with T1D and provide recommendations for next steps to develop effective interventions for this population across the

[a] Department of Family Medicine and Public Health Sciences, Wayne State University School of Medicine; [b] Center for Translational Behavioral Medicine, Florida State University
* Corresponding author. Wayne State University, IBio Behavioral Health, 6135 Woodward Avenue, Detroit, MI 48202.
E-mail address: dellis@med.wayne.edu

Endocrinol Metab Clin N Am 52 (2023) 585–602
https://doi.org/10.1016/j.ecl.2023.05.002
endo.theclinics.com

translational research continuum. However, such studies have almost exclusively enrolled children from Black and Latinx communities, and therefore, the review is focused on these youth. The article begins with an overview of health disparities for Black and Latinx youth with T1D and risk factors that may account for these disparities because such findings are informative in identifying treatment targets that should be addressed in intervention research. Next, it provides a comprehensive review of studies testing interventions for Black and Latinx youth with T1D. It concludes with a discussion of the limitations of the current literature, including the small number of intervention studies conducted to date that have focused on minoritized youth, and provides recommendations to increase the development, testing, and dissemination of evidence-based interventions for communities with T1D at highest need.

Disparities in Health Outcomes

During the past 20 years, multiple studies have shown that Black and Latinx youth are at increased risk for suboptimal glycemic control.[5–7] For example, recent longitudinal data drawn from the SEARCH for Diabetes in Youth study[8] found that Black and Latinx youth were more likely to have worsening trajectories of HbA1c during a 9-year period than White youth. Similar disparities have been documented in short-term diabetes complications rates, with Black and Latinx youth more likely to have diabetes-related hospitalizations for diabetic ketoacidosis (DKA) and episodes of severe hypoglycemia.[9,10] Studies investigating other important markers of overall health, such as cardiovascular status, also suggest elevated risk.[11,12] In the domain of psychosocial well-being, Black and Latinx youth with T1D may also be disproportionately impacted by diabetes. For example, diabetes distress is defined as the emotional burden of living with and managing diabetes.[13] At least one study found rates of diabetes distress to be significantly higher among both Black and Latinx youth than White youth.[14]

Although findings of health disparities for racial and ethnic minoritized youth may be due in part to the association between race/ethnicity and SES, studies attempting to disentangle these effects suggest that family income or social prestige accounts only in part for these disparities,[15] particularly among Black youth.[7] For Latinx youth, findings are less clear, with several studies showing that after accounting for SES, differences in diabetes health status between Latinx and White youth were no longer significant.[7,16]

FACTORS INFLUENCING DISPARITIES IN TYPE 1 DIABETES HEALTH OUTCOMES

The literature on family-level risks and assets for Black and Latinx youth with T1D is relatively sparse. However, existing studies suggest that Black and Latinx youth with T1D experience increased family-level risks, including higher rates of diabetes-related family conflict,[17,18] and lower parental supervision of adolescent diabetes management,[19] as compared with White youth. Family systems theory asserts that caregivers and children exert reciprocal influences on one another over time.[20,21] Caregivers of youth with T1D experience multiple stressors related to caring for a child with a complex chronic illness.[22,23] At least a study showed that Black caregivers in families with youth with T1D reported higher rates of diabetes-related distress than did White caregivers.[24] In turn, higher caregiver distress is associated with increased diabetes-related family conflict.[25]

Social determinants of health (SDoH), the social conditions and environment within which people are born, grow, live, work, and age,[26] have been of increased interest as critical factors that account for health disparities across disease conditions. Healthy

People 2030's model proposes 5 SDOH domains: economic stability, education access and quality, social and community contexts, neighborhoods and built environment, and health-care access and quality.[27] In the domain of health-care access and quality, medical management of T1D plays a significant role in health outcomes. Use of advanced diabetes treatment technologies such as continuous glucose monitors (CGM) and insulin pumps has become the standard of care due to the advantages they confer on diabetes health status.[28,29] However, inequities in their use have been ubiquitously demonstrated. One study showed that disparities in the rate of insulin pump use between White and Black youth widened from 2005 to 2019, with White youth more than twice as likely to use these devices[30] even after controlling for type of health care insurance (ie, public vs private). Several studies have also shown higher rates of discontinuation of CGM use among Black youth.[31]

The domain of social context, particularly discrimination, may also account for inequities in health outcomes for racial and ethnic minoritized youth with T1D. Health-care provider (HCP) perceptions of youth and family competence with regard to diabetes management play an important role in decisions regarding regimen intensification for youth with T1D.[32] Two recent studies by Addala and colleagues[33,34] demonstrated that the majority of HCPs caring for youth with T1D were more likely to recommend the use of advanced diabetes technology for youth who held private versus public insurance, whereas one of these studies also showed that one-third of HCPs were more likely to recommend such technology for White youth. Such studies indicate that implicit biases may influence HCP perceptions of youth or family competency to use advanced diabetes management technology, which in turn could affect prescribing decisions and youth access. Language-related barriers for Latinx families who are non-English speaking may also affect communication and relationships with HCPs,[35] which in turn may affect the diabetes management approach prescribed.

Finally, the impact of neighborhood conditions has also been explored. One study found associations between neighborhood disadvantage and glycemic control for Black, but not White, youth aged 5 to 20 years.[36] Another study using a sample of urban, low-income Black adolescents with T1D showed that level of neighborhood adversity was associated with glycemic control. This finding held even after controlling for family income, showing the independent effect of residing in low-resource neighborhoods. Bergmann and colleagues[37] showed that although readmissions for DKA 1 year after an index admission were associated with level of neighborhood disadvantage overall, Black youth were more likely than White youth living in similar levels of neighborhood disadvantage to experience readmissions.

In summary, Black and Latinx youth experience multiple risks that may account for disparities in T1D health outcomes. Next, we review intervention studies and consider the extent to which such studies have adequately targeted relevant risk factors, leveraged relevant assets, and/or tailored intervention content to meet the needs of these youth.

Selection of Intervention Studies Enrolling Black and Latinx Youth

The development of effective interventions to improve the health of youth with T1D requires researchers to conduct studies across the translational research spectrum, often referred to as T1–T4 (**Fig. 1**). In the context of intervention research, T1 studies are those feasibility, proof-of-concept or pilot studies that develop or test new treatments, whereas T2 studies are fully powered clinical trials that evaluate intervention efficacy under optimal conditions. T3 studies include effectiveness trials to test interventions in real-world settings, whereas T4 studies involve larger scale implementation of effective programs to assess broader public health impact. Both T3 and T4

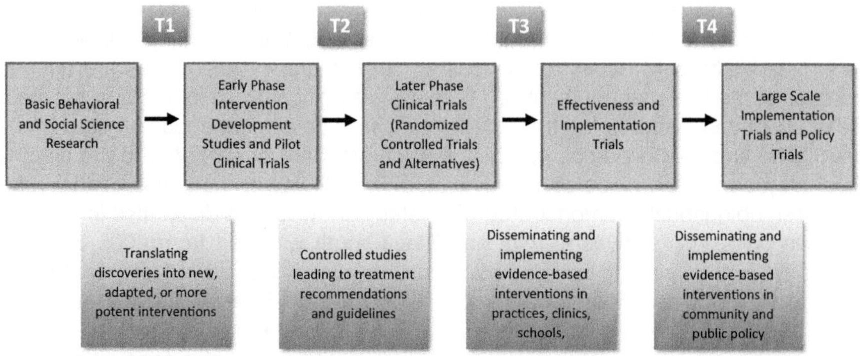

Fig. 1. Translational spectrum of intervention research. (*From* Naar S, Hudgens MG, Brookmeyer R, et al. Improving the Youth HIV Prevention and Care Cascades: Innovative Designs in the Adolescent Trials Network for HIV/AIDS Interventions. *AIDS Patient Care STDS.* 2019;33(9):388-398; with permission.)

studies often use implementation science methods, the study of how to best translate evidence-based practices to real-world settings.

For the present review, we included intervention studies at any stage of the T1–T4 continuum that primarily enrolled youth (at least 50% of the sample were aged younger than 18 years), focused on T1D (at least 50% of the sample with type 1 vs type 2 diabetes), and were conducted in the United States in the past 20 years. In addition, due to the extremely limited number of studies enrolling only racial and ethnic minoritized youth with T1D, we included any studies meeting the above criteria where at least 50% of sample was Black or Latinx. As noted earlier, we were not able to locate any intervention studies that enrolled substantial numbers (ie, >6%) of youth from Asian, Native American, or other minoritized populations. Because of the alignment of improvement science, which focuses on conducting systems-level work to improve the quality, safety, and value of health care, and implementation science,[38] we included one quality improvement study in our T4 studies where the focus was on improving health outcomes for Black or Latinx youth with T1D. We also included a second hospital-wide quality improvement study not solely focused on Black and Latinx youth because it specifically tested the effects of the improvement program on the subset of Black youth seen at the facility. **Table 1** shows the studies included in the review, along with the translational stage, study design, sample demographics, intervention characteristics, and intervention delivery location.

Review of Intervention Studies

T1 intervention studies: feasibility and pilot trials

The majority of studies identified for the review were T1 studies. Three studies used quasi-experimental designs to evaluate methods of improving standard medical care in clinic settings. The IMPACT study[39] used a single-arm clinical trial to assess whether the short-term use of a CGM provided by the youth's HCP influenced subsequent adoption and use of a personal CGM among non-CGM users. The sample consisted of 54% Black and Latinx youth. Youth attending a multidisciplinary diabetes clinic were provided with trial use of a CGM and/or smart phone if needed during a 10-day window and received standard education in CGM use as well as phone support during this period. At 3-to 6-month follow-up, 85% of youth reported wanting to use a personal CGM beyond the initial trial period. Of these, 76% (62% of the total

Table 1
Intervention studies reviewed across the translational continuum (T1–T4)

Author Year	Intervention Stage	Study Design	n	Race/Ethnicity	Household Income	Child Age	Intervention Content	Delivery Location
Ash et al,[42] 2019	T1	Single-arm clinical trial	18	39% Latinx 28% Black 28% White 6% Asian	US$20,000: 33% US$20–39,999: 22% ≥US$40,000: 34% Unknown: 11%	$\overline{\chi}$ = 14.1	MVPA plus diabetes education and parenting classes	University campus and community
Butler et al,[43] 2022	T1	Proof-of-concept	28	50% Latinx, 50% Black	Below US$60,000: 61% US$60,000 and above: 39%	$\overline{\chi}$ = 7.4	Group-based family teamwork intervention with tailored content plus peer coaches	Diabetes clinic
Ellis et al,[45] 2017	T1	Pilot randomized clinical trial	67	100% Black	Median: US$20,000–29,000	$\overline{\chi}$ = 12.1	Three-session, computer-delivered parenting intervention	Diabetes clinic and home
Ellis et al,[44] 2018	T1	Pilot randomized clinical trial	48	94% Black 2% White 4% "Other"	-	$\overline{\chi}$ = 18.2	MBSR, group-based CBT or diabetes support groups	University campus
Lin et al,[39] 2023	T1	Single-arm clinical trial	26	42% Black, 42% White, 12% Latinx 4% Native American	Below US$50,000: 43% US$50–100,000: 24% >US$100,000: 33%	$\overline{\chi}$ = 14.1	Participants provided with CGM for trial use during 10-d period; CGM education and support provided by diabetes clinic staff	Diabetes clinic
Palau-Collazo et al,[41] 2013	T1	Quasi-experimental	21	100% Latinx	-	$\overline{\chi}$ = 10.5	Spanish language diabetes clinic with all health-care providers required to be Spanish-speaking	Diabetes clinic

(*continued on next page*)

Table 1
(continued)

Author Year	Intervention Stage	Study Design	n	Race/Ethnicity	Household Income	Child Age	Intervention Content	Delivery Location
Pascual et al,[40] 2019	T1	Quasi-experimental	88	100% Latinx	-	<12 y $\bar{\chi}$ = 8.4 ≥ 12 y $\bar{\chi}$ = 14.6	SMA model with Spanish-speaking health-care providers; appointments followed by diabetes education groups structured by youth age	Diabetes clinic
Ellis et al,[48] 2007	T2	Randomized clinical trial	127	63% Black, 26% White, 11% "Other"	$\bar{\chi}$ = $27,950	$\bar{\chi}$ = 13.2	MST; intensive, family-based, multicomponent intervention	Home and community
Ellis et al,[49] 2012	T2	Randomized clinical trial	146	77% Black, 20% White 3% "Other"	-	$\bar{\chi}$ = 14.2	MST; intensive, family-based, multicomponent intervention	Home and community
Ellis et al,[59] 2019	T3	Pilot randomized effectiveness trial	48	79% Black 19% White 2% "Other"	$\bar{\chi}$ = $44,362	$\bar{\chi}$ = 14.3	Adapted version of MST; family-based, multicomponent intervention delivered by CHWs	Home and community
Ilkowitz et al,[57] 2016	T3	Quality improvement	Pre:523 Post:596	53% Latinx 47% Non-Latinx 24% Black 18% White 1% Asian 40% Multiracial 17% Unknown	-	Pre: $\bar{\chi}$ = 13.7 Post: $\bar{\chi}$ = 14.2	QI bundle to address multiple causes of DKA admission such as increasing the use of standardized DKA admissions by staff; provision of sick day education to all diabetes clinic patients;	Hospital-wide

							and addressing poor access to clinic appointments by increasing staffing	
Schmitt et al,[58] 2022	T3	Quality improvement	106	30% Black % Latinx not reported	-	-	QI bundle to increase patient CGM usage including weekly HCP reports on CGM utilization of scheduled patients; HCP education on benefits of CGM; providing patients with trial use of CGMs; and advocating for simplification of CGM coverage criteria for publicly insured patients with the state Medicaid agency	Hospital-wide

sample) had obtained a personal CGM but only 43% (35% of the total sample) continued to use the device. There were no significant improvements in HbA1c but there was a significant increase in youth-reported perceptions of CGM benefits.

A second quasi-experimental study used a pre-post design to evaluate the feasibility of a shared medical appointment (SMA) model for Spanish-speaking Latinx youth with T1D and their families.[40] The intervention included an individual meeting with the HCP for usual care, followed by a 2-hour meeting attended by 2 to 10 other families for diabetes education and support. Youth and caregivers participated in separate meetings. SMA visits alternated with usual care visits. Clinic staff were Spanish-speaking and program educational materials were translated into Spanish. Program retention was high at 77% after 2 years. For younger children, HbA1c improved significantly from baseline to the end of the second year of program implementation, as did uptake of insulin pump usage. Older youth did not show improvements in glycemic control but did significantly increase their use of insulin pumps.

A third quasi-experimental study compared 21 Latinx youth attending a newly established Spanish language clinic for pediatric patients with T1D with a matched sample of youth who attended the traditional diabetes clinic at the same site.[41] All staff in the Spanish language clinic spoke fluent Spanish and most were native speakers. The 2 groups of youth were matched by ethnicity, age of child, and duration of T1D. After 12 months, youth attending the Spanish language clinic group had a statistically significant decrease in HbA1c, whereas the comparison group had no significant change.

Two studies reported on feasibility approaches to evaluate behavioral interventions to address diabetes health. One study tested the use of moderate-to-vigorous physical activity (MVPA) among 18 adolescents with T1D and a sedentary lifestyle in a single-arm clinical trial.[42] Sixty-seven percent of the sample was non-White. The intervention involved group-based sessions that included 35 minutes of MVPA and 45 minutes of diabetes education on topic such as exercise, nutrition, and stress management. Group sessions were initially offered twice per week during 12 weeks but then reduced to once per week because only weekend sessions were feasible. Caregivers were offered parallel activities during the youth sessions. Enrollment was low because only 16% of those approached participated in the study, and only 56% completed the intervention. Among the 10 completers, endurance improved but MVPA and engagement in sedentary activities such as amount of daily screen time were unchanged in the overall sample.

Butler and colleagues[43] reported on the design phase, including cultural tailoring, of an intervention to increase collaborative diabetes management between Black and Latinx elementary-school aged children with T1D and their caregivers. An existing family-based intervention originally developed and tested with predominantly White adolescents with T1D was adapted in collaboration with community stakeholders and caregivers from the target population. Intervention modifications and strategies developed for the future clinical trial included "message mapping" for recruitment, development of cultural relevant intervention materials, using a group-based delivery format to increase peer support, inclusion of a peer leader as well as a professional to lead group sessions, and reducing the number of sessions in the program. However, quantitative findings from the trial were not presented in this study, and therefore, intervention efficacy could not be determined.

Finally, 2 studies used pilot randomized clinical trial designs to test behavioral interventions to improve diabetes health. One study targeted stress reduction as a mechanism for improving both diabetes management and glycemic control.[44] Youth aged 16 to 20 years (94% Black) were randomized to receive 1 of 3 group-based interventions: mindfulness-based stress reduction (MBSR), cognitive-behavioral therapy (CBT), or a diabetes support group. Each group received 9 treatment sessions. MBSR was found to significantly reduce self-reported stress at end of treatment and 3-month follow-up but no significant effects were found on diabetes management or glycemic control. Youth in the support group condition had significantly improved glycemic control but not diabetes management or stress. Findings supported the potential value of group-based interventions, including peer-support groups, for older adolescents.

The second pilot randomized controlled trial tested the effects of a 3-session, eHealth intervention delivered by a virtual avatar that aimed to increase daily parental supervision and monitoring of adolescent diabetes management among caregivers of young Black adolescents.[45] Intervention content was based on the information-motivation-behavior model[46] and was developed and beta-tested in collaboration with caregivers before the start of the clinical trial.[47] Adolescents and their primary caregiver were randomized to 1 of 3 arms: adolescent and parent eHealth intervention; adolescent education control and parent eHealth intervention; or adolescent and parent educational control. Recruitment and retention rates were high, as 71% of those approached were enrolled and 94% were retained through the end of the study. Caregivers in each study arm reported increases in knowledge of the need to engage in parental monitoring. The parent-only eHealth condition was the only arm where caregivers reported a trend to significant increase in parental monitoring of adolescent diabetes management. In this arm, adolescents also had significant improvements in HbA1c. A fully powered effectiveness-implementation hybrid trial of this intervention has recently been completed and preliminary results are further discussed in the section on T3/T4 studies below.

T2 intervention studies: fully powered clinical trials

Two T2 studies have been conducted that focused on predominantly racial and ethnic minoritized youth (ie, 74%–80% of these samples were non-White and most youth were Black).[48,49] In both of these studies, Ellis and colleagues conducted a randomized clinical trial to test the efficacy of Multisystemic Therapy, an intensive, home-based and community-based behavioral treatment, to improve diabetes management and glycemic control among adolescents with diabetes in suboptimal control. Multisystemic therapy (MST) has a number of characteristics that make it well suited for racial and ethnic minoritized youth. The intervention is based in social-ecological theory and includes the use of evidence-based interventions to address risk factors at multiple levels, including the individual adolescent (eg, providing tailored diabetes education), the family system (eg, increasing caregiver involvement in diabetes management), and the broader neighborhood and community systems within which the family is embedded (eg, improving family-HCP communication). In addition, the home-based and community-based approach allows barriers to accessing diabetes behavioral health care to be more efficiently managed. Finally, MST uses strength-based approaches to empower caregivers and youth by providing the skills and resources needed to manage diabetes. Results from these trials showed that adolescents receiving MST had significant improvements in diabetes management,[50] diabetes-related stress,[51] and health-related endpoints such as glycemic control[52] and DKA admissions[53] as compared with controls. Improvements in family relationships[54,55] and interactions with HCPs[56] were also reported for those receiving MST. Based on tests of moderators of MST's effectiveness to improve diabetes management and glycemic control, the intervention was found to be equally effective regardless of the youth's race/ethnicity.[48] However, because MST was not developed specifically for racial and ethnic minoritized adolescents with T1D, potential limitations of the intervention include the lack of engagement of stakeholders in intervention development or tailoring of the intervention content to fit the needs of these youth.

T3 and T4 intervention studies: effectiveness trials, implementation trials, and quality assurance programs

Given the dearth of T1 and T2 studies for Black and Latinx youth with T1D, and the associated lack of evidence-based interventions, T3/T4 studies for this population are in their infancy. Two of the studies reviewed were hospital-wide quality improvement studies, whereas one was a hybrid effectiveness-implementation trial. The first quality improvement study used a pre-post design to evaluate the effect of a program to reduce DKA admissions in an urban tertiary care pediatric hospital whose diabetes clinics serve a largely minoritized population (61% Latinx).[57] The quality improvement package included clinical (eg, increasing use of standardized DKA admissions criteria through routine team meetings), educational (eg, provision of sick day education to all diabetes clinic patients) and structural strategies (eg, addressing poor access to clinic appointments by increasing staffing). Admissions for the 3 years before and 2 years after implementation of the package were compared. Admissions with ketoacidosis per patient per year, length of stay, and unique patient 30-day DKA readmissions each decreased significantly from preimplementation to postimplementation.

A second quality improvement study addressed disparities in CGM use in a children's hospital located in the southeastern United States serving approximately 2000 youth with T1D.[58] The improvement program included increasing HCP awareness of CGM use among their patients by sending weekly reports of CGM utilization for scheduled patients; increasing HCP awareness of the benefits of CGM use through ongoing educational efforts; providing the opportunity for patients to engage in trial use of CGMs; and advocating for simplification of CGM coverage criteria for publicly insured patients with the state Medicaid agency. Prescription of a CGM by the HCP (defined as "access") was the primary outcome and was evaluated during the course of 13 months for youth with T1D managed in the facility. CGM access increased from 50% to 82%. Disparities in CGM access (defined as the difference in access between Whites and other groups) decreased from 18% to 6% for Blacks.

The only published randomized implementation trial to date was a pilot study of the delivery of MST, an evidence-based home and community intervention (see T2 interventions, above) by community health workers (CHWs) working for a federally qualified health center (FQHC).[59] The trial used an effectiveness-implementation design.[60] The intervention was adapted in collaboration with FQHC staff for delivery by CHWs before testing in the effectiveness clinical trial. Families (79% Black) were randomized to 6 months of the intervention, called reach for control (RFC) plus standard medical care or standard care (SC) only. A mixed-methods approach was used to evaluate implementation and effectiveness outcomes. Adolescents who received RFC had statistically significant and clinically meaningful improvements in HbA1c and reported significant improvements in quality of life from baseline to follow-up. The adolescents in standard medical care did not improve on any measure. Although delivery of the primary weekly family interventions sessions occurred at an acceptable rate, the number of brief follow-up sessions delivered was low due to CHW difficulties connecting with families to complete these. Evaluation of factors affecting successful implementation of the intervention by CHWs suggested that increasing CHW training in building relationships with adolescents and families, providing additional training to CHWs regarding T1D management and modification of the intervention dose were areas for future improvement.

Our research group recently completed a type 1 hybrid effectiveness-implementation trial (R01DK110075) conducted in 7 pediatric diabetes clinics across the United States that aimed to improve glycemic control in young Black adolescents with T1D; the study further evaluated the effectiveness of the eHealth intervention described above (see T1 studies) as well as barriers and facilitators to sustained use in tertiary diabetes care settings. Caregivers of young Black adolescents (N = 149) were randomized to receive the 3-session eHealth intervention via tablet computer during their child's regularly scheduled diabetes clinic visits during a 12-month period plus standard medical care or to SC alone. Adolescents assigned to the intervention group had a significant reduction in HbA1c from baseline to 6-month and 18-month follow-up of 0.53% ($P = .018$) and 0.83% ($P = .002$), respectively.

Analyses of barriers and facilitators to implementation of the intervention in pediatric diabetes clinics identified a number of relevant factors. In qualitative interviews, HCPs reported that it was important to support family involvement in adolescent diabetes care and that the psychosocial support provided through the intervention addressed a perceived gap in care in this area. Several HCPs also noted that an eHealth intervention was a good fit for the family-centered care approach of the institutions where the intervention was being tested (children's hospitals). Potential barriers identified by HCPs included the lack of available technology to deliver the intervention (eg, tablet computers), the potential for intervention delivery to disrupt of clinic flow and concerns regarding who would deliver the intervention. Solutions proposed included the use of electronic medical record (EMR) flags to identify eligible youth with T1D, creating marketing materials to engage families' interest in using the intervention and making the intervention available outside of the clinic.

DISCUSSION

The present review identified several areas of need, as well as promising directions, for the development of interventions to improve health equity in youth with T1D. First, the lack of intervention studies enrolling substantial numbers of racial and ethnic minoritized youth demonstrates the need to improve the use of effective recruitment strategies. Well-established recruitment strategies, such as developing trusting relationships with potential participants and the community as a whole, promoting cultural competency among recruitment staff, using convenient venues for recruitment and data collection (eg, home or community sites such as schools), and using a variety of recruitment strategies (eg, phone, contacts during clinical care appointments, outreach at community events),[61,62] need to be more routinely used in T1D clinical trials. Several of the studies reviewed tested interventions that were delivered either in the home or in community settings; such interventions may be a good fit for the needs of minoritized youth who may experience transportation or other barriers to participation in clinic-based interventions and may therefore increase recruitment success.

Although the lack of focus of any intervention studies on youth from Native communities or Asian/Pacific Islander youth may in part reflect the low base rate of T1D diagnosis in these groups, existing studies suggest they are also at heightened risk for diabetes-related disparities.[12,63] An increased focus on conducting studies to develop tailored intervention strategies for these youth and their families is clearly warranted.

A second area of need identified by the present review is the dearth of studies that tested culturally tailored interventions or used community-engaged approaches early in the development process. Approaches to cultural tailoring of interventions can include the design of intervention materials, translation of the intervention content, leveraging community members as part of intervention development or using cultural values and norms to provide context or meaning to the intervention.[64] The National Academy of Medicine has developed a comprehensive model of community engagement,[65] with measurable actions and outcomes. Integrating such benchmarks into future studies can improve authentic engagement. Despite the low number of studies to date, the recent use of community-engaged strategies to develop interventions and use of culturally tailored intervention content in several of the pilot studies included in the present review is promising. Preliminary evidence suggested that Spanish-language clinics, including those using a shared-medical appointment model, and brief interventions such as family-based, e-Health interventions hold the potential to increase the use of diabetes technologies such as CGM and to improve glycemic control for racial and ethnic minoritized youth with T1D.

The studies included in the present review largely provided either individual or family interventions consisted of content such as diabetes education and skills training, exercise, stress reduction, parent training, or family support. Early evidence from T1 studies suggests that offering brief trials of CGM may increase adolescent's perceptions that such devices would be helpful in their daily diabetes management. This approach was also supported in T3/T4 studies when used as one component of a quality improvement package. Findings from T2 studies also showed that multicomponent, family interventions were efficacious in improving multiple diabetes-specific endpoints, including hospital admissions for DKA. However, the growing literature on the critical influence of more distal risk factors such as access to resources and neighborhood conditions on the health of racial and ethnic minoritized youth with T1D demonstrates the importance of developing interventions to mitigate such risks. One of the T3/T4 studies reviewed found preliminary evidence that the use of CHWs

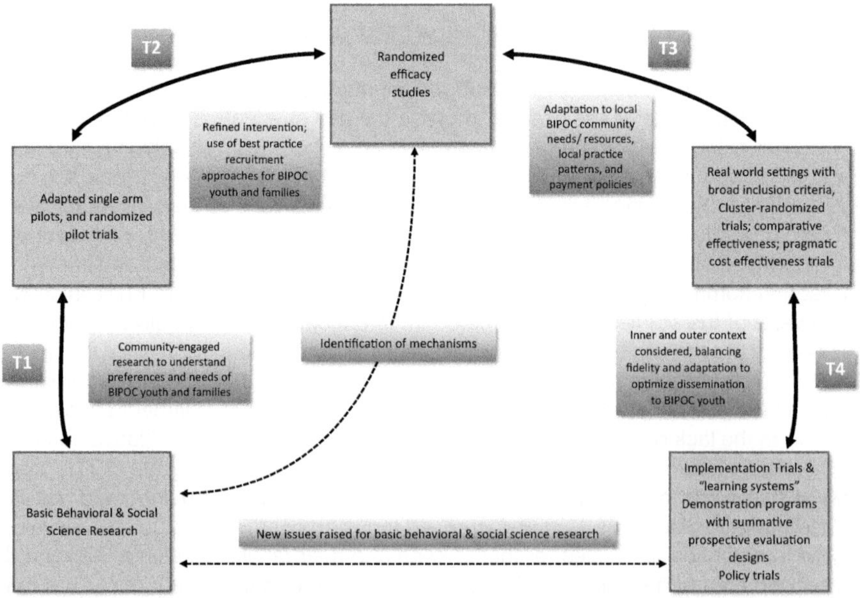

Fig. 2. New translational intervention model to guide research on racial and ethnic minoritized youth with T1D. (*From* Naar S, Hudgens MG, Brookmeyer R, et al. Improving the Youth HIV Prevention and Care Cascades: Innovative Designs in the Adolescent Trials Network for HIV/AIDS Interventions. AIDS Patient Care STDS. 2019;33(9):388-398; with permission.)

who addressed family resource needs as part of the intervention package could improve youth quality of life and glycemic control. Another showed that including advocacy with public insurance funders to ease restrictions that affected the use of CGM increased CGM access when used as part of a quality improvement program. More work to develop interventions that affect structural barriers to health equity is clearly needed. This includes the development and testing of antiracism interventions such as those beginning to be used in primary care contexts.[66]

In order to increase the pace at which evidence-based interventions are delivered to racial and ethnic minoritized youth with T1D, it may be necessary to reconsider the traditional step-wise approach to intervention development.[67] For example, efficacy-effectiveness hybrid trials retain the rigor of a "T2" efficacy trial while integrating "T3" effectiveness components such as the recruitment of diverse participants and utilizing real-world intervention strategies.[68] Another important direction to increase the pace at which effective interventions to improve health equity are delivered to racial and ethnic minoritized youth is to address inequities through quality improvement studies. The Type 1 Diabetes Exchange QI initiative uses a learning health system approach with continuous quality-improvement methods that leverage electronic medical record data to improve T1D health outcomes.[69] Health equity goals include measuring relevant metrics through electronic records, addressing provider bias and institutional racism, and developing dashboards with health equity benchmarks that can be continuously updated and monitored. Such efforts will likely also strengthen future T1D health equity.

SUMMARY

In conclusion, new models that do not rely on traditional phased approaches may be needed to accelerate the pace of developing efficacious interventions for racial and ethnic minoritized youth with T1D and ensuring widespread dissemination and adoption of such interventions. **Fig. 2** shows a modified approach to translational intervention development for racial and ethnic minoritized youth with T1D that reflects the need to accelerate the pace of implementation of effective interventions for this population while ensuring that community-driven priorities are considered. In this model, translational stages each inform one another and need not follow in a prescribed sequence. Rather, the need for scientific rigor in intervention development is addressed by using novel experimental designs in earlier stages of the intervention continuum,[70] recognizing taxonomies of implementation strategies that allow comparisons across studies and explaining implementation variability,[71] and using improvement science strategies to systematically address care quality.[38] Continued collaborative efforts from clinicians and researchers working equitably with community members are needed to improve the quality of T1D intervention science across the translational research spectrum.

CLINICS CARE POINTS

- Offering brief trials of CGM use with structured support from clinic staff may help increase perception of benefits from advanced diabetes technology among minoritized youth, which in turn may improve personal device adoption and longer term use.
- Improving cultural competency of pediatric diabetes care by offering language-congruent clinics or a SMA model may improve health outcomes for Latinx youth.

- Because evidence supports the potential of CHWs to improve health outcomes in minoritized youth with T1D, their use as clinic extenders should be considered when youth experience suboptimal glycemic control.
- Advocacy by HCPs to simplify the coverage criteria and/or approval process for the use of advanced diabetes technology required by public insurance programs can serve an important role in overcoming structural barriers to optimal diabetes management that increase health disparities.

DISCLOSURE

The authors have no conflicts of interest to disclose. Funding for the research was provided in part by NIDDK R01DK110075 and NIMHD R01MD017404

REFERENCES

1. Pettitt DJ, Talton J, Dabelea D, et al. Prevalence of diabetes in U.S. youth in 2009: the SEARCH for diabetes in youth study. Diabetes Care 2014;37(2):402–8.
2. Lipman TH, Levitt Katz LE, Ratcliffe SJ, et al. Increasing incidence of type 1 diabetes in youth: twenty years of the Philadelphia Pediatric Diabetes Registry. Diabetes Care 2013;36(6):1597–603.
3. Lado JJ, Lipman TH. Racial and Ethnic Disparities in the Incidence, Treatment, and Outcomes of Youth with Type 1 Diabetes. Endocrinol Metab Clin North Am 2016;45(2):453–61.
4. Keenan ME, Berlin KS, Cook JL, et al. Predictors of HbA1c Trajectories in Predominantly Black Adolescents With Type 1 Diabetes. J Pediatr Psychol 2021; 46(3):241–50.
5. Redondo MJ, Libman I, Cheng P, et al. Racial/Ethnic Minority Youth With Recent-Onset Type 1 Diabetes Have Poor Prognostic Factors. Diabetes Care 2018;41(5): 1017–24.
6. Wang JT, Wiebe DJ, White PC. Developmental trajectories of metabolic control among White, Black, and Hispanic youth with type 1 diabetes. J Pediatr 2011; 159(4):571–6.
7. Willi SM, Miller KM, DiMeglio LA, et al. Racial-ethnic disparities in management and outcomes among children with type 1 diabetes. Pediatrics 2015;135(3): 424–34.
8. Kahkoska AR, Shay CM, Crandell J, et al. Association of Race and Ethnicity With Glycemic Control and Hemoglobin A(1c) Levels in Youth With Type 1 Diabetes. JAMA Netw Open 2018;1(5).
9. Lipman TH, Smith JA, Patil O, et al. Racial disparities in treatment and outcomes of children with type 1 diabetes. Pediatr Diabetes 2021;22(2):241–8.
10. Cengiz E, Xing D, Wong JC, et al. Severe hypoglycemia and diabetic ketoacidosis among youth with type 1 diabetes in the T1D Exchange clinic registry. Pediatr Diabetes 2013;14(6):447–54.
11. Faulkner MS, Quinn L, Fritschi C, et al. Heart Rate Variability and Cardiorespiratory Fitness in Non-Hispanic Black Versus Non-Hispanic White Adolescents With Type 1 Diabetes. J Cardiovasc Nurs 2019;34(5):372–9.
12. Rodriguez BL, Dabelea D, Liese AD, et al. Prevalence and Correlates of Elevated Blood Pressure in Youth with Diabetes Mellitus: The Search for Diabetes in Youth Study. J Pediatr 2010;157(2):245–51.e241.
13. Skinner TC, Joensen L, Parkin T. Twenty-five years of diabetes distress research. Diabet Med : a journal of the British Diabetic Association 2020;37(3):393–400.

14. Fegan-Bohm K, Minard CG, Anderson BJ, et al. Diabetes distress and HbA1c in racially/ethnically and socioeconomically diverse youth with type 1 diabetes. Pediatr Diabetes 2020;21(7):1362–9.
15. Tremblay ES, Liu E, Laffel LM. Health Disparities Likely Emerge Early in the Course of Type-1 Diabetes in Youth. J Diabetes Sci Technol 2022;16(4):929–33.
16. Mello D, Wiebe D. The Role of Socioeconomic Status in Latino Health Disparities Among Youth with Type 1 Diabetes: a Systematic Review. Curr Diabetes Rep 2020;20(11):56.
17. Caccavale LJ, Weaver P, Chen R, et al. Family Density and SES Related to Diabetes Management and Glycemic Control in Adolescents With Type 1 Diabetes. J Pediatr Psychol 2015;40(5):500–8.
18. Nicholl MC, Valenzuela JM, Lit K, et al. Featured Article: Comparison of Diabetes Management Trajectories in Hispanic versus White Non-Hispanic Youth with Type 1 Diabetes across Early Adolescence. J Pediatr Psychol 2019;44(6):631–41.
19. Ellis DA, Templin TN, Podolski CL, et al. The parental monitoring of diabetes care scale: development, reliability and validity of a scale to evaluate parental supervision of adolescent illness management. J Adolesc Health 2008;42(2):146–53.
20. McHale SM, Amato P, Booth A. Emerging methods in family research. New York (NY): Springer Science and Business Media; 2013.
21. Queen TL, Butner J, Wiebe DJ, et al. A micro-developmental view of parental well-being in families coping with chronic illness. J Fam Psychol 2016;30(7): 843–53.
22. Carcone AI, Ellis DA, Naar-King S. Linking caregiver strain to diabetes illness management and health outcomes in a sample of adolescents in chronically poor metabolic control. J Dev Behav Pediatr 2012;33(4):343–51.
23. Whittemore R, Jaser S, Chao A, et al. Psychological experience of parents of children with type 1 diabetes: a systematic mixed-studies review. Diabetes Educ 2012;38(4):562–79.
24. Evans MA, Weil LEG, Shapiro JB, et al. Psychometric Properties of the Parent and Child Problem Areas in Diabetes Measures. J Pediatr Psychol 2019;44(6): 703–13.
25. Jaser SS, Linsky R, Grey M. Coping and psychological distress in mothers of adolescents with type 1 diabetes. Matern Child Health J 2014;18(1):101–8.
26. Solar O, Irwin A. A conceptual framework for action on the social determinants of health. WHO Document Production Services; 2010.
27. U.S. Department of Health and Human Services OoDPaHP. Healthy People 2030. ,Available at: https://health.gov/healthypeople/objectives-and-data/social-determinants-health. Accessed 1 12, 2023.
28. Sherr JL, Schoelwer M, Dos Santos TJ, et al. ISPAD Clinical Practice Consensus Guidelines 2022: Diabetes technologies: Insulin delivery. Pediatr Diabetes 2022; 23(8):1406–31.
29. Tauschmann M, Forlenza G, Hood K, et al. ISPAD Clinical Practice Consensus Guidelines 2022: Diabetes technologies: Glucose monitoring. Pediatr Diabetes 2022;23(8):1390–405.
30. Lipman TH, Willi SM, Lai CW, et al. Insulin Pump Use in Children with Type 1 Diabetes: Over a Decade of Disparities. J Pediatr Nurs 2020;55:110–5.
31. Lai CW, Lipman TH, Willi SM, et al. Racial and Ethnic Disparities in Rates of Continuous Glucose Monitor Initiation and Continued Use in Children With Type 1 Diabetes. Diabetes Care 2021;44(1):255–7.

32. Valenzuela JM, La Greca AM, Hsin O, et al. Prescribed regimen intensity in diverse youth with type 1 diabetes: role of family and provider perceptions. Pediatr Diabetes 2011;12(8):696–703.
33. Addala A, Hanes S, Naranjo D, et al. Provider Implicit Bias Impacts Pediatric Type 1 Diabetes Technology Recommendations in the United States: Findings from The Gatekeeper Study. J Diabetes Sci Technol 2021;15(5):1027–33.
34. Odugbesan O, Addala A, Nelson G, et al. Implicit Racial-Ethnic and Insurance-Mediated Bias to Recommending Diabetes Technology: Insights from T1D Exchange Multicenter Pediatric and Adult Diabetes Provider Cohort. Diabetes Technol Ther 2022;24(9):619–27.
35. Gandhi KK, Baranowski T, Anderson BJ, et al. Psychosocial aspects of type 1 diabetes in Latino- and Asian-American youth. Pediatr Res 2016;80(3):347–55.
36. Coulon SJ, Velasco-Gonzalez C, Scribner R, et al. Racial differences in neighborhood disadvantage, inflammation and metabolic control in black and white pediatric type 1 diabetes patients. Pediatr Diabetes 2017;18(2):120–7.
37. Bergmann KR, Nickel A, Hall M, et al. Association of Neighborhood Resources and Race and Ethnicity With Readmissions for Diabetic Ketoacidosis at US Children's Hospitals. JAMA Netw Open 2022;5(5):e2210456.
38. Koczwara B, Stover AM, Davies L, et al. Harnessing the Synergy Between Improvement Science and Implementation Science in Cancer: A Call to Action. J Oncol Pract 2018;14(6):335–40.
39. Lin T, Manfredo JA, Illesca N, et al. Improving Continuous Glucose Monitoring Uptake in Underserved Youth with Type 1 Diabetes: The IMPACT Study. Diabetes Technol Ther 2023;25(1):13–9.
40. Pascual AB, Pyle L, Nieto J, et al. Novel, culturally sensitive, shared medical appointment model for Hispanic pediatric type 1 diabetes patients. Pediatr Diabetes 2019;20(4):468–73.
41. Palau-Collazo MM, Rose P, Sikes K, et al. Effectiveness of a spanish language clinic for Hispanic youth with type 1 diabetes. Endocr Pract 2013;19(5):800–4.
42. Ash GI, Joiner KL, Savoye M, et al. Feasibility and safety of a group physical activity program for youth with type 1 diabetes. Pediatr Diabetes 2019;20(4):450–9.
43. Butler AM, Hilliard ME, Fegan-Bohm K, et al. Peer-support intervention for African American and Latino parents to improve the glycemic control trajectory among school-aged children with type 1 diabetes: A pilot and feasibility protocol. Contemp Clin Trials 2022;116:106739.
44. Ellis DA, Carcone AI, Slatcher R, et al. Efficacy of mindfulness-based stress reduction in emerging adults with poorly controlled, type 1 diabetes: A pilot randomized controlled trial. Pediatr Diabetes 2019;20(2):226–34.
45. Ellis D, Carcone A, Ondersma S, et al. Brief computer-delivered intervention to increase parental monitoring in families of african American adolescents with type 1 diabetes: a randomized controlled trial. Telemedicine and e-Health; 2017.
46. Fisher WA, Fisher JD, Harman J. The information-motivation-behavioral skills model: A general social psychological approach to understanding and promoting health behavior. In: Suls J, Wallston KA, editors. Social psychological foundations of health and illness. Oxford (United Kingdom): Blackwell Publishing Ltd; 2003. p. 82–106.
47. Carcone AI, Ellis DA, Naar S, et al. Enhancing parental motivation to monitor African American adolescents' diabetes care: Development and beta test of a brief computer-delivered intervention. JMIR research protocols 2014;3(3):e43.

48. Ellis DA, Templin T, Naar-King S, et al. Multisystemic therapy for adolescents with poorly controlled type I diabetes: Stability of treatment effects in a randomized controlled trial. J Consult Clin Psychol 2007;75(1):168–74.
49. Ellis D, Naar-King S, Chen X, et al. Multisystemic Therapy Compared to Telephone Support for Youth with Poorly Controlled Diabetes: Findings from a Randomized Controlled Trial. Ann Behav Med 2012;44(2):207–15.
50. Ellis DA, Frey MA, Naar-King S, et al. Use of multisystemic therapy to improve regimen adherence among adolescents with type 1 diabetes in chronic poor metabolic control: a randomized controlled trial. Diabetes Care 2005;28(7): 1604–10.
51. Ellis DA, Frey MA, Naar-King S, et al. The effects of multisystemic therapy on diabetes stress among adolescents with chronically poorly controlled type 1 diabetes: findings from a randomized, controlled trial. Pediatrics 2005;116(6): e826–32.
52. Ellis DA, Naar-King S, Chen X, et al. Multisystemic therapy compared to telephone support for youth with poorly controlled diabetes: findings from a randomized controlled trial. Ann Behav Med 2012;44(2):207–15.
53. Ellis D, Naar-King S, Templin T, et al. Multisystemic therapy for adolescents with poorly controlled type 1 diabetes: reduced diabetic ketoacidosis admissions and related costs over 24 months. Diabetes Care 2008;31(9):1746–7.
54. Ellis D, Yopp J, Templin T, et al. Family mediators and moderators of treatment outcomes among youths with poorly controlled Type 1 diabetes: Results from a randomized controlled trial. J Pediatr Psychol 2006;32(2):194–205.
55. Naar-King S, Ellis DA, Idalski A, et al. Multisystemic therapy decreases parental overestimation of adolescent responsibility for type 1 diabetes management in urban youth. Fam Syst Health 2007;25(2):178–89.
56. Carcone AI, Ellis DA, Chen X, et al. Multisystemic Therapy Improves the Patient-Provider Relationship in Families of Adolescents with Poorly Controlled Insulin Dependent Diabetes. J Clin Psychol Med Settings 2015;22(2–3):169–78.
57. Ilkowitz JT, Choi S, Rinke ML, et al. Pediatric Type 1 Diabetes: Reducing Admission Rates for Diabetes Ketoacidosis. Qual Manag Health Care 2016;25(4): 231–7.
58. Schmitt J, Fogle K, Scott ML, et al. Improving Equitable Access to Continuous Glucose Monitors for Alabama's Children with Type 1 Diabetes: A Quality Improvement Project. Diabetes Technol Ther 2022;24(7):481–91.
59. Ellis DA, Carcone AI, Naar-King S, et al. Adaptation of an Evidence-Based Diabetes Management Intervention for Delivery in Community Settings: Findings From a Pilot Randomized Effectiveness Trial. J Pediatr Psychol 2019;44(1): 110–25.
60. Curran GM, Bauer M, Mittman B, et al. Effectiveness-implementation Hybrid Designs Combining Elements of Clinical Effectiveness and Implementation Research to Enhance Public Health Impact. Med Care 2012;50(3):217–26.
61. Cui Z, Seburg EM, Sherwood NE, et al. Recruitment and retention in obesity prevention and treatment trials targeting minority or low-income children: a review of the clinical trials registration database. Trials 2015;16:564.
62. Ellis DA, Rhind J, Carcone AI, et al. Optimizing Recruitment of Black Adolescents into Behavioral Research: A Multi-Center Study. J Pediatr Psychol 2021;46(6): 611–20.
63. Malik FS, Sauder KA, Isom S, et al. Trends in Glycemic Control Among Youth and Young Adults With Diabetes: The SEARCH for Diabetes in Youth Study. Diabetes Care 2022;45(2):285–94.

64. Torres-Ruiz M, Robinson-Ector K, Attinson D, et al. A Portfolio Analysis of Culturally Tailored Trials to Address Health and Healthcare Disparities. Int J Environ Res Public Health 2018;15(9):1859.
65. Aguilar-Gaxiola S, Ahmed SM, Anise A, et al. Assessing Meaningful Community Engagement: A Conceptual Model to Advance Health Equity through Transformed Systems for Health: Organizing Committee for Assessing Meaningful Community Engagement in Health & Health Care Programs & Policies. NAM Perspect 2022;2022:1–12.
66. Hassen N, Lofters A, Michael S, et al. Implementing Anti-Racism Interventions in Healthcare Settings: A Scoping Review. Int J Environ Res Public Health 2021;18(6):1–15.
67. Glasgow RE, Lichtenstein E, Marcus AC. Why don't we see more translation of health promotion research to practice? Rethinking the efficacy-to-effectiveness transition. Am J Publ Health 2003;93(8):1261–7.
68. Kathleen MC, Bruce JR. Bridging the Gap: A Hybrid Model to Link Efficacy and Effectiveness Research in Substance Abuse Treatment. Psychiatr Serv 2003;54(3):333–9.
69. Ebekozien O, Mungmode A, Odugbesan O, et al. Addressing type 1 diabetes health inequities in the United States: Approaches from the T1D Exchange QI Collaborative. J Diabetes 2022;14(1):79–82.
70. Klasnja P, Hekler EB, Shiffman S, et al. Microrandomized trials: An experimental design for developing just-in-time adaptive interventions. Health Psychol 2015;34s(0):1220–8.
71. Powell BJ, Waltz TJ, Chinman MJ, et al. A refined compilation of implementation strategies: results from the Expert Recommendations for Implementing Change (ERIC) project. Implement Sci 2015;10(1):21.

Diabetes Care in Humanitarian Settings

Sylvia Kehlenbrink, MD[a,*], Kiran Jobanputra, MBChB, MPH[b], Amulya Reddy, MD, MPH[b], Philippa Boulle, MBBS, MPH, DHTM[c], Apoorva Gomber, MBBS, MD, MPH[d], Rachel Nugent, PhD[e], Vinod Varma, MD, MA[f], Anna T. Nakayama, MSc, RD, LDN, ANutr[g], Tom Ellman, MBChB, MRCP[h]

KEYWORDS

• Diabetes • Humanitarian setting • Humanitarian crises • Health equity

KEY POINTS

- Despite the growing diabetes epidemic and record-high numbers of forcibly displaced populations globally, both of which predominantly affect lower- and middle-income countries, health systems are often unable to maintain diabetes care during humanitarian emergencies.
- Diabetes services delivered by humanitarian nongovernmental organizations vary significantly, and there are no predefined minimum standards, services, or operating procedures for diabetes care in a crisis.
- Humanitarian crises are often characterized by population displacement, destruction of social networks, loss of livelihoods, food insecurity, violence, human rights abuses, and a high prevalence of mental health disorders which further impact diabetes management and increase risk for people with diabetes.
- Despite noncommunicable diseases, including diabetes, dominating the global burden of disease, they are arguably the most underfunded issue in global health.

[a] Division of Endocrinology, Diabetes and Hypertension, Brigham and Women's Hospital, 221 Longwood Avenue RFB-2, Boston, MA 02115, USA; [b] Médecins Sans Frontières, Chancery Exchange, Lower Ground Floor, 10 Furnival Street, London EC4A 1AB, UK; [c] Médecins Sans Frontières, Route de Ferney 140, Geneva 1202, Switzerland; [d] Division of Global Health Equity, Brigham and Women's Hospital, Center for Integration Science, 75 Francis Street, Boston MA 02115, USA; [e] Department of Global Health, University of Washington, 3980 15th Avenue Northeast, Seattle, WA 98195, USA; [f] The Global Fund to Fight AIDS, Tuberculosis and Malaria, Chemin du Pommier 40, 1218 Grand-Saconnex, Geneva, Switzerland; [g] International Alliance for Diabetes Action, 101 South Hanley Road, Suite 800, Saint Louis, MO 63105, USA; [h] Médecins Sans Frontières, 9th Floor, Zurich House, 70 Fox Street, Marshalltown, Johannesburg 2001, South Africa
* Corresponding author.
E-mail address: skehlenbrinkoh@bwh.harvard.edu

Endocrinol Metab Clin N Am 52 (2023) 603–615
https://doi.org/10.1016/j.ecl.2023.05.010 endo.theclinics.com

INTRODUCTION

In 2022 over 100 million people globally had been forcibly displaced from their homes as a result of conflict and violence.[1] Over 80% are hosted in lower- and middle-income countries (LMICs). In addition, on average 200 million people are affected by natural disasters each year.[2] One in every 23 people worldwide needs emergency assistance to survive.[3] The dramatic impact of conflicts and climate-related natural disasters, coupled with major trends such as water scarcity, population growth, and urbanization, are leaving people vulnerable and in need of humanitarian assistance for decades, and in some cases, for generations.[4] In such contexts, people living with chronic diseases such as diabetes are particularly vulnerable.[5]

In parallel, over the past few decades the global burden of disease and the consequent health needs of those facing humanitarian crisis have changed. The prevalence of diabetes has skyrocketed and currently affects over half a billion people worldwide.[6] Diabetes ranks among the top 10 causes of death globally with over 80% of those affected living in LMICs. However, access to diabetes care in many LMIC contexts is highly inequitable, and is not included in Universal Health Coverage (UHC) benefits packages in many countries.[7,8] Free access to diagnosis or care in low-income countries is rare, such that even outside humanitarian settings over 50% of adults with diabetes in these countries are unaware of their status and only 50% of those who are diagnosed are on treatment; there are large gaps all along the diabetes care cascade in LMICs.[6,7] Thus, diabetes constitutes a global crisis in its own right.

Humanitarian crises increase the risk of negative health outcomes through numerous mechanisms: violence and insecurity, mass displacement, deterioration of living conditions, impoverishment, health service disruption, and reduced availability of human and financial resources.[9] Those who most come to harm tend to have multiple vulnerabilities. This was particularly evident during the COVID-19 pandemic where diabetes was associated with more severe infection and poorer outcomes, especially among socially vulnerable populations, and care was most affected by essential service disruption in LMICs.[10–12] Moreover, hazards and vulnerabilities are unequally distributed in humanitarian crises, and health services are rarely allocated according to need. In high- and middle-income settings where diabetes care is typically available outside the context of crisis, the impact of a humanitarian emergency may be seen in the temporary disruption of those services. By contrast, in low-resource settings where pre-crisis diabetes care may have been weak or lacking, demand during a crisis may be less apparent, but arguably the needs are as great or greater.

Despite the increasing prevalence of diabetes in populations experiencing humanitarian crisis, along with evidence that people living with diabetes (PLWD) are at higher risk for poor outcomes in a crisis, health systems are often unable to maintain comprehensive diabetes care during crisis (even where diabetes is included in the UHC benefits package). Furthermore, diabetes care is often not integrated in humanitarian health interventions. This is despite the inclusion of NCDs on the 2030 Agenda for Sustainable Development adopted by the United Nations (UN) General Assembly in 2015 which characterized noncommunicable diseases (NCDs) as a threat to development and a cause and consequence of poverty and inequality.[13] The 2023 Agenda includes a vision for global solidarity with people in fragile environments, with the imperative to "leave no one behind." This critical gap was outlined in the Boston Declaration in 2019 which was signed by over 60 signatories with humanitarian assistance missions and included a joint agenda to work toward over the coming years, updated in 2022 to reflect the changing global landscape and current needs.[5,14]

We here describe 4 factors that have contributed to the inequities and lack of diabetes inclusion in humanitarian programmes: (1) evolving paradigms in humanitarian health care, (2) complexities of diabetes service provision in humanitarian settings, (3) social and cultural challenges, and (4) lack of NCD financing. In addition, we outline opportunities and possible interventions to address these challenges and improve diabetes care among crisis-affected populations.

Evolving Paradigms in Humanitarian Health Care

The medical humanitarian response has tended primarily to focus on identification of immediate needs and application of a public health approach to maximize benefit for the largest number of people. Given competition for scarce resources in humanitarian emergencies, a disease or need where the lowest number needed to treat results in the highest number of lives saved or suffering averted takes priority. A model developed for late Cold War crises meant relatively young populations were displaced to refugee camps, whereas interventions aimed to minimize excess mortality from infectious diseases and malnutrition became the norm.[15] The original 1997 Sphere standards—a set of universal minimum standards for humanitarian response that are widely used by humanitarian agencies—contained almost no mention of NCDs. This gap has been addressed in recent editions, reflecting the gradually growing awareness among humanitarian agencies of the importance of NCDs.[16] The original focus on infectious diseases resulted in humanitarian actors being slow to adapt to the epidemiological shift toward increasing chronic diseases, disability, and diseases of aging. This failure is exacerbated by the "expediency" culture of humanitarian response, which has tended to assume needs rather than invest the time required to consult with the affected communities to learn about needs.

Because of the changing nature and geographical distribution of conflict, as well as overlapping climate- and environment-related chronic emergencies in recent decades, crises have become increasingly protracted. In 2018, the average length of humanitarian crises with UN-coordinated responses was over 9 years, up from 5.2 years in 2014.[17] In 2021, the UN Refugee Agency reported over 70% of refugee situations are protracted.[18] People affected are more often in countries with higher baseline income and life expectancy, internally displaced and living in noncamp urban and rural settings where health interventions are more difficult to implement.[18] Corresponding priority health needs have changed, with NCDs being prevalent, but without an adapted humanitarian health response that includes chronic care.

For many humanitarian agencies, care for NCDs is harder to include in humanitarian response planning. The addition of diabetes care requires an investment in capacity building that not only takes time but must consider the existing health system, with which programmes must integrate. NCD services are more likely to be sustained post-emergency in settings where care existed pre-crisis, compared to settings where chronic disease services were not routinely available previously. This raises issues of equitable care for displaced and host populations and the value of a time-limited response to a chronic need in acute emergencies if services are not sustained post-emergency. It is important to deliver a standard of care that takes into consideration both the need for equity between host and displaced populations and the implications of closure of services if they cannot be sustained beyond the short or medium term. As with HIV, the provision of critical and life-saving care, including insulin, should never be denied on the basis that long-term sustainability may not be feasible.

The nature of inequality and inaccessibility of diabetes services in LMICs means that success for access in humanitarian emergencies will be contingent on broader regional and country-level achievements in NCD care. Therefore, concerted effort is needed to render host country health systems capable of supporting people with diabetes and other NCDs, and to ensure emergency preparedness plans include care for diabetes and are integrated with health system planning as part of Disaster Risk Reduction (DRR).[19]

Diabetes and other NCDs have not yet garnered the level of civil society engagement and the related high levels of donor and government commitment that continues to propel successes in communicable diseases, such as HIV. This partially explains the lack of diabetes services and fatalism regarding the possibility of long-term continuity care for chronic diseases as part of the humanitarian response. However, some HIV programmes are starting to include care for comorbid diabetes and increase attention to NCDs, as people living with HIV have an increased life expectancy and require diabetes and other NCD services.

There is currently some momentum in awareness raising of the issues PLWD face. The World Health Organization (WHO) Global Diabetes Compact Forum involves expert patients with lived experience and the NCD Alliance is developing regional influence. These need to be supported while increased independent patient-led advocacy and activism are made a priority to ensure equity in diabetes care.

Complexities of Providing Diabetes Care in Crises

The design of diabetes services in humanitarian crises depends on multiple factors including pre-existing services, acuity of the crisis, and resource availability.[20] In the acute emergency phase, maintaining continuity of care for people already on treatment is priority, in particular for people for whom treatment interruption could be life-threatening or cause significant avoidable suffering, such as those with type 1 diabetes.[20] This requires identification of those individuals and ensuring access to care. However, baseline diabetes prevalence data and national or facility-based registries are often unavailable and standardized indicators and data collection tools for NCDs are lacking, making identification and continuity of care for these individuals challenging.[21] Moreover, diabetes services delivered by non-governmental organizations vary significantly and there are no pre-defined minimum standards, services, or operating procedures for diabetes care in a crisis. The lack of routine inclusion of diabetes care (including insulin) in emergency preparedness or response plans means diabetes-related supplies can be absent, delayed, or incomplete.[22]

Continuous access to medical supplies for the ongoing management of diabetes in crisis settings is often challenging. Supply chain interruptions and physical obstacles are frequently immediate barriers to care, as was recently seen following onset of the crises in Ukraine and Turkey. The WHO Interagency Emergency Health Kit (IEHK) contains essential medicines and supplies for a population of 10,000 for a 3-month period in the immediate aftermath of a crisis. Insulin was not included in the kit until 2016. Subsequently, the WHO developed an NCD kit to complement the IEHK that includes oral hypoglycemics, human insulin, as well as syringes, lancets, and glucose strips.[23,24] Although this kit has been an important asset in recent humanitarian emergencies, challenges have included significant supply chain delays and limited staff training in NCD management.[25] Maintaining a continuous supply of medications, diagnostics, and regular medical review for migrants and refugees on the move remains challenging. Therefore, the importance of self-management is nowhere more pertinent than crisis contexts. However, the provision of therapeutic patient education and empowerment is easily deprioritized in emergency responses.

Insulin supply, management, and storage in humanitarian settings are particularly difficult. In lower resource settings, there may be a pre-existing lack of access to insulin and diagnostics in the public sector. Moreover, the insulin provided by humanitarian agencies in an emergency and that in common use prior to the crisis may be different. Patients may need to change from the medications they were taking previously to those that are available and move from patented to generic drugs. Therefore, information for health care staff and people with diabetes regarding switching between insulin and other therapies plays a critical role while responding to humanitarian crises. In recognition of this, switching guides have been created and translated into different languages relevant to recent emergencies.[26] However, standardized guidance and education on the management of insulin in acute emergencies are lacking. In addition, since refrigeration is often limited in low-resource and humanitarian settings and some organizations do not dispense insulin for home use when it is not available, the storage of insulin in these settings remains a critical barrier to care.[20] Diabetes diagnostics, such as HbA1c and glucose self-monitoring, are not routinely available in emergencies, although the use of simple point of care devices by humanitarian organizations has proven beneficial for rapid assessment and adaptation of care.[22]

Diabetes care provision in high-resource settings is a multidisciplinary endeavor, with a variety of specialists, health care workers, and allied care providers to support patients with medication guidance, follow-up, and self-management needs. In low-resource settings, this team of health care workers is less commonly available and care, if available, is often concentrated in centralized services where specialists or medical doctors are available; treatment of acute complications relies on a robust referral system. In recent years, WHO has prioritized support for countries to develop "Emergency Care Systems Frameworks," which ensure rapid access to secondary care for diabetes complications, yet these frameworks remain relatively weak in low-resource settings.[27] Furthermore, in the context of humanitarian crisis, referral systems frequently break down, and as a result the provision of all diabetes care tends to rely on primary health care services.[28]

The usual absence of diabetes-experienced staff in humanitarian settings has meant that the organization of care, task distribution, and support to medical teams must be deliberately adapted per setting. Humanitarian organizations can work with staff including generalist doctors or clinical officers, nurses, lay health promotion staff, or community health workers.[20] Therefore, training and support to staff at various levels is vital. Telemedicine or remote expert support can help with complex care management if access to specialists is otherwise not available.[29] The role of PLWD in providing care in crisis settings is just starting to be explored, to provide more adapted, person-centered care that empowers those in need, and better equips them for the unfortunate reality of potentially tenuous care continuity.

Social and Cultural Issues

Diabetes management and outcomes are known to be strongly influenced by the social determinants of health.[12,30] These are profoundly impacted by humanitarian crises that are often characterized by population displacement, destruction of social networks, loss of livelihoods, insecurity, violence, and human rights abuses.[31] In addition, the impact of humanitarian crises on mental health further undermines diabetes control.[32] These factors and the associated disruption to daily routines impact the ability of PLWD to self-manage their diabetes care.[33]

Food insecurity and irregular dietary patterns can increase the risk of hypoglycemia and potentially prove fatal for people with type 1 diabetes.[28] Unreliability in the quantity and quality of available food, food scarcity, and rationing of insulin for extended durations results in sub-optimal glycemic control and has been shown to increase the risk of hyperglycemic emergencies like diabetes ketoacidosis.[34] Traditional food assistance programmes were developed to treat undernutrition in acute emergencies and typically provide a low-diversity diet that do not meet the dietary needs of people with diabetes and have the potential to exacerbate NCDs.[35–37] Indeed, individuals with diabetes have reported their fear that diet adherence will be the biggest obstacle to follow their diabetes treatment plan.[38]

At baseline, diabetes has a pervasive image problem and negative attitudes and social stigma are often overlooked when providing care.[39,40] People with diabetes often experience stigma, disproportionately affecting those with higher body mass index (BMI) and poor blood glucose control,[41–43] due to cultural aspects and psychological mechanisms such as blame, fear, and disgust.[44] In displaced populations, an individual's understanding of diabetes, perceptions of quality of care, and legal barriers influence health-seeking behaviors. People diagnosed after onset of a crisis have been shown to have less knowledge about diabetes and less medication adherence than those diagnosed before displacement, posing a significantly higher risk for complications.[45–47] Lack of reliable diabetes understanding, community support, and knowledge about diabetes may result in delays in seeking medical care.[38] Community relationship building, education, and psycho-social exercises within peer group settings after a crisis can offer opportunities for building safe spaces to support PLWD in humanitarian settings.[38,48]

Financing of Diabetes Among Crisis-Affected Populations

NCDs receive under 2% of all global health financing despite them dominating the global burden of disease.[49] This has remained roughly stable while overall global health financing has increased continuously over 2 decades, with a record high amount in 2021, thanks to almost $40 billion spent for COVID-19 over the first 2 years of the pandemic.[50,51] In general, donor funding disproportionately goes towards infectious diseases, such as the Ebola outbreak in 2014 ($1.6 billion), HIV/AIDS ($39 billion since 1990), and tuberculosis ($5.5 billion since 2005) (**Table 1**).

What these responses share is the perceived immediacy of the infectious disease threat to wider populations, especially to populations in high-income countries that are the source of most donor assistance for health. Thus, donor funding for global health is heavily skewed toward communicable diseases, even in humanitarian emergencies where access to government-provided health care is unavailable or erratic.[52] Lack of funding means that without access to free health care people living with NCDs either receive no care or impoverish themselves trying to pay for it.

While emergencies also command immediate attention and financial resources, the above bias remains. Neglect of NCDs in favor of infectious risks is compounded by a focus on children and young people in emergencies rather than older adults, and on acute rather than chronic needs. A recent study showed that of all Overseas Development Aid (ODA) disbursed for health between 2010 and 2019 for around 35 million internally displaced persons, less than 1% of the total went to NCDs.[53]

Beginning in 2014, global health security (GHS) emerged as a subfield of global health that convenes public and private stakeholders to strengthen the response to infectious disease threats, including the now-chronic conditions of HIV/AIDS and tuberculosis.[54] GHS recognizes a constellation of risks that lies at the intersection of global health and global emergencies including the impacts of climate change and other slow-developing disasters, as NCDs have been called.[55] GHS offers prevention, detection, response, and containment actions that can eliminate or manage those risks. These risks affect everyone but, as COVID-19 showed, often affect those with underlying chronic conditions most acutely. Although GHS thus affords a broad view of health threats–well beyond the disease-specific approach–agenda-setting

Table 1
Development assistance for health by focus and program area, 1990–2021

Health Focus Areas and Program Areas	1990	1995	2000	2005	2010	2015	2021[a]	Total
HIV/AIDS	464	940	1528	5685	11,773	8974	9911	39,275
Malaria	54	89	168	760	2153	1895	2438	7557
Noncommunicable diseases	54	104	184	171	459	611	1081	2663
Newborn and child health	747	1339	1978	3381	5123	8484	9498	30,548
Other infectious diseases[b]	191	172	1184	833	1636	3913	24,006	31,934
Reproductive and maternal health	1937	2654	2800	2504	4504	5225	5301	24,926
Health system strengthening/sector-wide approaches	1698	2201	2938	3998	6091	5093	7212	29,232
Tuberculosis	24	75	142	544	1636	1365	2033	5818
Other health focus areas[c]	2931	3470	2654	5082	4173	4264	5933	28,507
Unallocable	452	394	333	132	169	0	0	1479
Total	8550	11,436	13,908	23,086	37,707	39,823	67,412	201,922

This table disaggregates development assistance for health earmarked for HIV/AIDS; maternal, newborn, and child health; malaria; tuberculosis; other infectious diseases; noncommunicable diseases; and health systems strengthening and sector-wide approaches.

All figures are in millions of US dollars.

[a] 2021 estimates are preliminary.

[b] Includes antimicrobial resistance, COVID-19, Ebola, Health systems strengthening, Zika, and Other.

[c] "Other health focus areas" captures development assistance for health for which we have health focus area information, but which is not identified as being allocated to any of the health focus areas listed. Contributions from remaining channels are shown as unallocable by disease.

Source: Institute for Health Metrics Evaluation. Used with permission.

Box 1
Needs and opportunities to improve diabetes care in humanitarian settings

1. Strengthen integration of diabetes in humanitarian preparedness and response plans.
   - Enhance collaboration between health systems and health emergency communities to enable joint planning for emergency preparedness and care continuity.
   - Strengthen coordination among humanitarian organizations by ensuring expert representation on NCDs within the WHO emergency coordinating body (Health Cluster).
   - Assess the capacity of referral systems (from primary to secondary care) to safely manage hyperglycemic emergencies, and if necessary, strengthen the system by applying the WHO "Emergency Care System Framework" or equivalent approaches.
   - Improve integration of diabetes and NCDs in health needs assessments, emergency preparedness, health information, and surveillance systems, ensuring they function in the context of humanitarian crises.
   - Conduct operational evaluations and implementation research to routinely adapt programmes based on lessons learned to ensure programs continue to meet the needs of PLWD.
   - Ensure that the essential components of the continuum of care for diabetes that are part of UHC benefits packages are guaranteed for people living in humanitarian emergencies.
2. Develop simplified operational and clinical care approaches for diabetes to ensure service sustainability.
   - Develop and pilot an operational toolkit for diabetes and NCDs in emergencies, including guidance across the continuum of care. Integrate lessons from COVID-19 for maintaining essential services, detection of emergency cases, remote screening, and health education.
   - Create a Minimum Initial Service Package for Diabetes with standard operating procedures for assessing and facilitating the availability of essential medications and diagnostics and establish a predefined and coordinated set of activities to manage diabetes that are implemented at the onset of every emergency.
   - Learn from the example of HIV care provision in humanitarian settings, applying models of care that use task sharing between different levels of health care workers, include staff dedicated to patient education and support, have a system for follow-up and include a cohort approach to data collection and analysis.
   - Develop simplified and standardized clinical guidance for ready use by less experienced clinicians implementing diabetes care in acute emergencies to support use of the WHO NCD Emergency Kits, including the storage of insulin without refrigeration.
   - Ensure the prioritization, procurement and deployment of essential, safe, affordable, and effective diabetes medicines, technologies, and supplies, and maintain continuity of medication in emergencies including through the development and use of the NCD kit.
3. Increase awareness of social aspects of diabetes care (including in crises) and involvement of PLWD.
   - Strengthen advocacy for inclusion of PLWD in design and development of diabetes services, through existing initiatives such as the WHO Global Diabetes Compact Forum. Support and prioritize independent patient-led advocacy and activism.
   - Develop and promote culturally appropriate diabetes self-management, education, and support approaches to enhance coping and resilience among vulnerable populations.
   - Integrate mental health and psychosocial support and diabetes care services in humanitarian settings; improve awareness efforts to address and reduce social stigma and promote empowering and respectful language.
   - Develop an emergency preparedness toolkit and education for PLWD to be implemented prior to an emergency.
   - Tailor health promotion advice and patient support to available food resources, adapt food assistance policies to include NCDs, and increase food diversity in food assistance programmes.
4. Work with donors to raise awareness of diabetes needs in crisis and develop sustainable funding models.

- Work with planning departments to establish mechanisms to secure adequate contingency and transitional financing for NCD care in emergency response and recovery, including ongoing funding of successful NCD pilot programmes that were initiated in emergencies.
- Advocate for greater funding for NCDs in building health system resilience.
- Work with donors and humanitarian organizations to shift their perspectives to a longer-term, more flexible assessment and response to needs. For example, blending funding streams from global health and emergency response agencies to ensure diabetes services that are implemented as part of the emergency response are continued beyond the acute emergency phase.

on GHS rarely refers to chronic NCDs and more often tends to align with a narrower, Western perspective of health security, as described above.[56]

The security risks that arise when fragile or under-resourced health systems face sudden new challenges call for donors and government financing to take a broader view of what health security really means. The economic costs and productivity losses created by a large and growing NCD burden are well documented, including increased severity of infectious disease as well as costly-to-treat sequelae and complications of chronic diseases.[57] Many of the issues highlighted for an effective infectious risk response—surveillance, workforce development, laboratories, risk communication, and financing—are identical to what is called for in a stronger NCD response.[56] Whether in stable or humanitarian settings and regardless of immediate perceived pandemic threats, global health security cannot be achieved through a narrow focus on funding only the most obvious infectious disease threats.

WHAT IS NEEDED?

We have described 4 factors that have contributed to the inequities and neglect of diabetes care in humanitarian emergencies. PLWD will continue to lack health equity in crisis contexts unless the drivers of these deficits are addressed. In **Box 1** we highlight opportunities to overcome each challenge.

SUMMARY

The ongoing lack of diabetes care in humanitarian contexts has created persistent health disparities for PLWD that will continue to worsen unless action is taken. By assessing the factors that drive the heath inequities, we find that there are pragmatic and attainable opportunities to provide essential diabetes care in humanitarian settings. It is critical to prioritize equitable care to PLWD and uphold the humanitarian imperative, that without exception, action should be taken to prevent or alleviate suffering from crises.

CLINICS CARE POINTS

- Health system contingency planning needs to include mechanisms to ensure that the essential components of the continuum of care for diabetes can be maintained during periods of service disruption (whether due to workforce issues, outbreaks, or humanitarian emergencies).
- Disaster management/public health emergency departments, as well as international agencies responding to health and humanitarian emergencies, should ensure diabetes is

included in emergency preparedness plans, emergency health assessments, and initial service packages for humanitarian response.

- Simplified and standardized clinical guidance for ready use by less experienced clinicians implementing diabetes care in acute emergencies is needed.
- To ensure crisis preparedness and mitigate risk, providing education on prevention and management of treatment interruptions for people living with diabetes prior is critical.
- Blending funding streams from global health and emergency response agencies is needed to ensure diabetes services that are implemented as part of an emergency response are continued beyond the acute emergency.

DISCLOSURE

The authors declare no conflicts of interests. All views are personal and do not represent those of the author's affiliated institutions.

REFERENCES

1. United Nations High Commissioner for Refugees (UNHCR). More than 100 million people are forcibly displaced. 2022. Available at: https://www.unhcr.org/refugee-statistics/insights/explainers/100-million-forcibly-displaced.html. (Accessed January 13, 2023).
2. Human cost of disasters: an overview of the last 20 years (2000-2019). Geneva, Switzerland: Centre for Research on the Epidemiology of Disasters and UN Office for Disaster Risk Reduction; 2019.
3. United Nations Office for the Coordination of Humanitarian Affairs (OCHA) , 2023 Global humanitarian overview presentation: under-secretary-general for humanitarian affairs and emergency relief coordinator martin griffiths, 2022, Geneva, Switzerland.
4. Forced displacement: refugees, asylum seekers and internally displaced persons (IDPs). Brussels, Belgium: European Civil Protection and Humanitarian Aid Operations; 2022.
5. Kehlenbrink S, Jobanputra K, Ansbro É, et al. A framework for improving diabetes care in humanitarian emergencies. Lancet Diabetes Endocrinol 2023;11(3):146–9.
6. International Diabetes Federation. IDF Diabetes Atlas, 10th Edition. Brussels, Belgium: 2021. Available at: https://www.diabetesatlas.org.
7. Flood D, Seiglie JA, Dunn M, et al. The state of diabetes treatment coverage in 55 low-income and middle-income countries: a cross-sectional study of nationally representative, individual-level data in 680 102 adults. The Lancet Healthy Longevity 2021;2(6). e340-e51.
8. Manne-Goehler J, Geldsetzer P, Agoudavi K, et al. Health system performance for people with diabetes in 28 low- and middle-income countries: a cross-sectional study of nationally representative surveys. PLoS Med 2019;16(3):e1002751.
9. Health in Humanitarian Crises Centre Report 2017. London, UK: London School of Hygiene and Tropical Medicine; 2017.
10. The impact of the COVID-19 pandemic on noncommunicable disease resources and services: results of a rapid assessment. Geneva, Switzerland: World Health Organization; 2020.
11. Sosa-Rubí SG, Seiglie JA, Chivardi C, et al. Incremental risk of developing severe COVID-19 among mexican patients with diabetes attributed to social and health care access disadvantages. Diabetes Care 2020;44(2):373–80.

12. Seiglie JA, Nambiar D, Beran D, et al. To tackle diabetes, science and health systems must take into account social context. Nat Med 2021;27(2):193–5.
13. United Nations. (2016). *Transforming our world: the 2030 Agenda for Sustainable Development.* Available at: https://sdgs.un.org/2030agenda. (Accessed June 5, 2023).
14. Kehlenbrink S, Jaacks LM, Aebischer Perone S, et al. Diabetes in humanitarian crises: the Boston Declaration. Lancet Diabetes Endocrinol 2019;7(8):590–2.
15. Spiegel PB, Checchi F, Colombo S, et al. Health-care needs of people affected by conflict: future trends and changing frameworks. Lancet 2010;375(9711):341–5.
16. The Sphere handbook: humanitarian charter and minimum standards in humanitarian response. Geneva, Switzerland: Sphere Association; 2018.
17. United Nations Office for the Coordination of Humanitarian Affairs (OCHA). (2018) US$21.9 billion needed in 2019 as average length of humanitarian crises climbs. Available at: https://www.unocha.org/story/us219-billion-needed-2019-average-length-humanitarian-crises-climbs. (Accessed February 23, 2023).
18. United Nations High Commissioner for Refugees (UNHCR) (2022), Global trends: forced displacement in 2021. Geneva, Switzerland.
19. Bello OBA, Pizzaro P. Planning for disaster risk reduction within the framework of the 2030 Agenda for Sustainable Development. Geneva, Switzerland: United Nations ECLAC; 2021.
20. Kehlenbrink S, Ansbro É, Besançon S, et al. Strengthening diabetes care in humanitarian crises in low- and middle-income settings. J Clin Endocrinol Metab 2022;107(9):e3553–61.
21. Kehlenbrink S, Smith J, Ansbro É, et al. The burden of diabetes and use of diabetes care in humanitarian crises in low-income and middle-income countries. Lancet Diabetes Endocrinol 2019;7(8):638–47.
22. Kehlenbrink S, Mahboob O, Al-Zubi S, et al. An inter-humanitarian agency study of diabetes care and surveillance in humanitarian settings. Lancet Diabetes Endocrinol 2022;10(3):159–62.
23. Slama S, Lee J, Aragno M, et al. The development of the noncommunicable diseases emergency health kit. East Mediterr Health J 2018;24(1):92–8.
24. World Health Organization. Noncommunicable diseases kit (NCDK) 2022. 2022. Available at: https://www.who.int/emergencies/emergency-health-kits/non-communicable-diseases-kit-2022. (Accessed February 23, 2023 2023).
25. Kiapi L, Alani AH, Ahmed I, et al. Assessment of the non-communicable diseases kit for humanitarian emergencies in Yemen and Libya. BMJ Glob Health 2022; 7(Suppl 5):e006621.
26. Insulin Switching Guides. 2022. Available at: https://diabetesdisasterresponse.org/urkriane. (Accessed April 21, 2022).
27. World Health Organization, WHO emergency care system framework, 2018. Available at: https://www.who.int/publications/i/item/who-emergency-care-system-framework. (Accessed February 27, 2023).
28. Boulle P, Kehlenbrink S, Smith J, et al. Challenges associated with providing diabetes care in humanitarian settings. Lancet Diabetes Endocrinol 2019;7(8):648–56.
29. Santé Diabète. Response strategy covid-19-diabetes 2020. Grenoble, France.
30. Hill-Briggs F, Adler NE, Berkowitz SA, et al. Social determinants of health and diabetes: a scientific review. Diabetes Care 2020;44(1):258–79.
31. World Health Organization (2008), Social determinants of health in countries in conflict: a perspective from the Eastern Mediterranean Region, Available at: https://applications.emro.who.int/dsaf/dsa955.pdf. (Accessed June 5, 2023).

32. Gyawali B, Harasym MC, Hassan S, et al. Not an 'either/or': Integrating mental health and psychosocial support within non-communicable disease prevention and care in humanitarian response. J Glob Health 2021;11:03119.
33. Balabanova D, McKee M, Koroleva N, et al. Navigating the health system: diabetes care in Georgia. Health Policy Plan 2009;24(1):46–54.
34. Nhoung HK, Goyal M, Cacciapuoti M, et al. Food insecurity and insulin use in hyperglycemic patients presenting to the emergency department. West J Emerg Med 2020;21(4):959–63.
35. Carruth L, Ateye MJ, Nassir A, et al. Diabetes in a humanitarian crisis: atypical clinical presentations and challenges to clinical- and community-based management among Somalis in Ethiopia. Global Publ Health 2020;15(6):828–39.
36. Food and nutrition handbook. Rome, Italy: World Food Programme; 2018.
37. Hawkes C, Ruel MT, Salm L, et al. Double-duty actions: seizing programme and policy opportunities to address malnutrition in all its forms. Lancet 2020; 395(10218):142–55.
38. Murphy A, Biringanine M, Roberts B, et al. Diabetes care in a complex humanitarian emergency setting: a qualitative evaluation. BMC Health Serv Res 2017; 17(1):431.
39. Palmer T, Waliaula C, Shannon G, et al. Understanding the lived experience of children with type 1 diabetes in kenya: daily routines and adaptation over time. Qual Health Res 2022;32(1):145–58.
40. Hunt D, Lamb K, Elliott J, et al. A WHO key informant language survey of people with lived experiences of diabetes: Media misconceptions, values-based messaging, stigma, framings and communications considerations. Diabetes Res Clin Pract 2022;193:110109.
41. Liu NF, Brown AS, Folias AE, et al. Stigma in people with type 1 or type 2 diabetes. Clin Diabetes 2017;35(1):27–34.
42. Schabert J, Browne JL, Mosely K, et al. Social stigma in diabetes. The Patient - Patient-Centered Outcomes Research 2013;6(1):1–10.
43. Inagaki S., Matsuda T., Muramae N., et al., Diabetes-related shame among people with type 2 diabetes: an internet-based cross-sectional study, *BMJ Open Diabetes Res Care*, 10 (6), 2022, e003001.
44. Major B, O'Brien LT. The social psychology of stigma. Annu Rev Psychol 2005;56: 393–421.
45. Elliott JA, Das D, Cavailler P, et al. A cross-sectional assessment of diabetes self-management, education and support needs of Syrian refugee patients living with diabetes in Bekaa Valley Lebanon. Conflict Health 2018;12:40.
46. Elliott JA, Abdulhadi NN, Al-Maniri AA, et al. Diabetes self-management and education of people living with diabetes: a survey in primary health care in Muscat Oman. PLoS One 2013;8(2):e57400.
47. el-Shazly M, Zaki A, Nicolucci A. Care-related risk factors for chronic diabetic complications in developing countries: a case from Egypt. Publ Health 2002; 116(5):289–96.
48. Shahin YKAKA, Zeidan W, Harries AD, et al. Clinical audit on the provision of diabetes care in the primary care setting by United Nations Relief and Works Agency for Palestine Refugees in the Near East (UNRWA). J Diabetes Mellitus 2015;5: 12–20.
49. Jailobaeva K, Falconer J, Loffreda G, et al. An analysis of policy and funding priorities of global actors regarding noncommunicable disease in low- and middle-income countries. Global Health 2021;17(1):68.

50. Institute for Health Metrics and Evaluation (IHME). Financing global health 2021: global health priorities in a time of change. Seattle, Washington.
51. Global Burden of Disease Health Financing Collaborator N. Global investments in pandemic preparedness and COVID-19: development assistance and domestic spending on health between 1990 and 2026. Lancet Global Health 2023;11(3): e385–413.
52. Shiffman J, Shawar YR. Framing and the formation of global health priorities. Lancet 2022;399(10339):1977–90.
53. Roberts B, Ekezie W, Jobanputra K, et al. Analysis of health overseas development aid for internally displaced persons in low- and middle-income countries. Journal of Migration and Health 2022;5:100090.
54. Gostin LO, Meier BM, Stocking B. Developing an Innovative Pandemic Treaty to Advance Global Health Security. J Law Med Ethics 2021;49(3):503–8.
55. United Nations (2011). Non-communicable diseases deemed development challenge of 'epidemic proportions', In: *Political declaration adopted during landmark general assembly summit*, 2011, United Nations Meetings Coverage and Press Releases. Available at: https://press.un.org/en/2011/ga11138.doc.htm. (Accessed June 5, 2023).
56. Kostova D, Richter P, Van Vliet G, et al. The role of noncommunicable diseases in the pursuit of global health security. Health Secur 2021;19(3):288–301.
57. NCD Countdown 2030 collaborators, NCD Countdown 2030: efficient pathways and strategic investments to accelerate progress towards the Sustainable Development Goal target 3.4 in low-income and middle-income countries, Lancet, 399 (10331), 2022, 1266–1278.

Equity in Obesity Review

Karla N. Kendrick, MD, MPH[a,*], Kevin J. Bode Padron, BS[b,c], Nichola Z. Bomani, BA[b,d], Jashalynn C. German, MD[e], Dennis D. Nyanyo, BA[a,f,g], Brenda Varriano, MD, MSc[h], Lucy Tu[i,j], Fatima Cody Stanford, MD, MPH, MPA, MBA[k]

KEYWORDS

• Obesity • Health equity • Disparities • Social determinants of health • Health policy

KEY POINTS

- Obesity is a chronic disease with multifactorial causes that disproportionately affects minoritized populations and those of lower socioeconomic status.
- Health-care providers should recognize bias and stigma as barriers patients face in seeking care for managing obesity.
- Body mass index should be used as a screening rather than a diagnostic tool to allow clinicians to better assess health risks at varying weight thresholds.

INTRODUCTION

The prevalence of obesity has dramatically increased in recent decades. The 2019 Global Burden of Disease Study demonstrated an age-standardized prevalence of obesity of 14% worldwide, nearly triple that of obesity in 1975.[1] Alongside the dysregulation of adipocytes and energy homeostasis,[2] obesity contributes to chronic comorbidities of cardiovascular disease, diabetes, osteoarthritis, obstructive sleep apnea, and profound disability.[3,4] This results in increased costs and strain on health-care systems[5,6] but also negatively affects the quality of life of billions.

[a] Beth Israel Lahey Health, Winchester Hospital Weight Management Center; [b] Massachusetts General Hospital Neuroendocrine and Pituitary Tumor Clinical Center, 100 Blossom Street, Cox Building Suite 140, Boston, MA 02114, USA; [c] Duke University School of Medicine, DUMC 2927, 40 Duke Medicine Circle, 124 Davison Building, Durham, NC 27710, USA; [d] Case Western Reserve University School of Medicine, 9501 Euclid Avenue, Cleveland, OH 44106, USA; [e] Duke Division of Endocrinology, Metabolism, and Nutrition, 200 Trent Drive, Baker House, DUMC Box 3021, Durham, NC 27710, USA; [f] Harvard Medical School, 25 Shattuck Street, Boston, MA 02115, USA; [g] Harvard Kennedy School of Government, 79 John F. Kennedy Street, Cambridge, MA 02138, USA; [h] Mass-General Hospital, 55 Fruit Street, Boston, MA 02114, USA; [i] Department of Sociology, Harvard University, 33 Kirkland Street, Cambridge, MA, USA; [j] Department of History of Science, Harvard University, 1 Oxford St #371, Cambridge, MA, USA; [k] Massachusetts General Hospital MGH Weight Center, 50 Staniford Street, Suite 430, Boston, MA 02114, USA

* Corresponding author. 200 Unicorn Park Drive, Suite 401, Woburn, MA 01801.
E-mail address: karlankendrick@gmail.com

Endocrinol Metab Clin N Am 52 (2023) 617–627
https://doi.org/10.1016/j.ecl.2023.05.003
endo.theclinics.com

Rates of obesity have increased similarly in the United States,[7] with disproportionate influences on women, Black, Latino, lesbian, gay, bisexual, transgendered, queer (LGBTQ+), and lower income individuals.[8] Despite prevention efforts on behalf of hospital systems, schools, and governments,[9,10] as well as novel breakthroughs in the medical management of obesity,[11] obesity rates continue to increase, with worsening disparity.[12] Viewing obesity from a lens of racial, ethnic, and socioeconomic equity is critical to both understanding and mitigating the inequalities in the prevalence and treatment of obesity. Care from an equity-informed perspective wields the potential to improve communication, patient–provider relationships, the patient agency in care,[13] and long-term health outcomes.[14]

In this review, we describe the current state of racial, ethnic, and socioeconomic disparities within the prevalence and medical management of obesity in the United States. We also address the structural and societal contributions to this disparity, including access to care, environmental challenges, social stigma, economics, and the discriminatory origins of body mass index (BMI) as a defining metric for obesity. Current efforts to advance equity in clinical obesity care are highlighted in a multilevel approach, with recommendations from individual, community, and policy perspectives.

BACKGROUND

Obesity is a growing epidemic that disproportionately affects specific populations. Non-Hispanic Black and Hispanic adults, people with low socioeconomic status, inhabitants of rural areas, and those identifying as LGBTQ face higher burdens of obesity and obesity-related complications.[15] The prevalence of obesity in the United States continues to grow. Data from the 2017 to 2018 National Health and Nutrition Examination Survey indicated an estimated 42.4% of US adults aged 20 years and older had obesity, an increase from 33.7% in 2007 to 2008.[16] Non-Hispanic Black adults had the highest prevalence of obesity (49.6%) compared with Asian adults (17.4%), non-Hispanic White (42.2%), and Hispanic (44.8%) adults.[16] Additionally, non-Hispanic Black adults had the highest prevalence of severe obesity (BMI $\geq$40) at an estimated 13.8% compared with a prevalence of 9.2% across all races.[16]

These differences in obesity prevalence are preventable and influenced by factors within and outside the health-care system.[17] Disparities within the health-care systems include differences in access to care or discrepancies in the likelihood of receiving specific treatments. The cornerstones of obesity management include lifestyle interventions focused on diet, physical activity, pharmacologic therapy, and surgical interventions. It has been shown that racial/ethnic minoritized individuals and individuals of lower socioeconomic status (SES) face unique circumstances that make reaching healthy eating and physical activity goals challenging, such as a higher likelihood of living in food deserts and being likely to be engaged in organized sports or have means to pursue other recreational physical activities.[18] The number of Federal Drug Administration-approved pharmacotherapies to manage obesity continues to grow. Research investigating the equitable use of obesity medications is scarce with inconsistent findings. Some studies have demonstrated lower utilization among Hispanic/Latino and non-Hispanic Black populations compared with non-Hispanic Whites populations. In contrast, other studies have not found racial/ethnic disparities.[19–21] In regards to SES, those working full time may be more likely to discuss obesity medications with health-care providers compared with those with part time employment (Arterburn 2013).[22] Furthermore, the lack of coverage for obesity medications disproportionately affects those of lower SES because Medicare strictly excludes coverage, and only 15 traditional Medicaid programs nationwide provide coverage for obesity medication (Stephenson 2022).[23] Despite racial and ethnic minoritized groups having higher rates of obesity than White populations, Black and Hispanic populations are less likely to undergo bariatric surgery, an intervention shown to yield remarkable health improvement and reduce mortality.[18,24–26] When they undergo bariatric surgery, Black and Hispanic individuals and those of low income also have less weight loss compared with White individuals (Zhao 2021).[27]

Disparities related to race and ethnicity are apparent not only in obesity prevalence but also in the rates of obesity-related comorbidities, including hypertension, diabetes, and arthritis.[28] Additionally, the lifetime risk for cardiovascular disease and metabolic abnormalities such as dyslipidemia is increased disproportionally in Black and Hispanic populations compared with White counterparts.[29] Genetics, dietary and physical activities, psychological factors, stress, income, and discrimination have all previously been identified as factors resulting in higher obesity and obesity-related complications among Hispanic and non-Hispanic Black populations.[18]

MECHANISMS OF INEQUITIES

Structural Mechanisms

The mechanisms that drive health inequities in obesity prevalence and care are diverse, evolving, and interdependent and include structural and individual factors. First, the origins of BMI, widely used to define obesity, are rooted in life insurance data collected among mostly White men from the 1930s to the 1950s that was used to determine the risk of mortality and certain diseases due to weight and height differences.[30] This raises concern about the generalizability of thresholds that define obesity and one's risk of adverse conditions because of weight.[31] For example, a Japanese individual can be healthier at a lower BMI, and Polynesian individuals can be healthier at higher BMIs.[32–34] At similar BMIs, non-Hispanic Black individuals tend to carry more weight in their limbs than trunks compared with non-Hispanic White individuals,[35] which may affect the risk of metabolic syndrome.

Neighborhood and built environmental factors also play a role in disparities in obesity. Racial and ethnic minoritized individuals often experience residential segregation and live in low-income neighborhoods in poor proximity to health-care facilities, which limits access to health-care resources.[36] Residential segregation experienced by minoritized communities results from "redlining," a directive from the Federal Housing Administration following the Great Depression that led neighborhood appraisals to consider residents' race in determining the investment risk. Decades of community disinvestment, lack of opportunities for home ownership, and wealth accumulation among racial and ethnic minoritized communities are upstream social determinants of health implicated in obesity and its adverse health outcomes.[37]

Racial discrimination likely contributes to disparities in obesity as well. In one study, self-reported racism has been shown to correlate with negative health behaviors, thus increasing the risk for obesity, smoking, and binge drinking.[38] Moreover, this study reported that patients experiencing racism were less likely to be up to date with health screenings, especially if they were of African American ancestry, compared with Latinos and Whites.[38] Internalized racism has been correlated with negative interactions with other individuals and health professionals.[39–41] Those experiencing the highest levels of discrimination are at a higher risk of stress, obesity, and complications of obesity such as diabetes.[39–41]

Low-income neighborhoods are also associated with obesity due to other factors such as walkability, access to healthy foods, and safety. Low neighborhood safety discourages walking and outdoor activity.[42] Low-income neighborhoods are also located closer to fast-food restaurants and convenience stores, thus limiting access to healthy food options.[43] A study of the New York City food environment and walkability by Rundle and colleagues[44] revealed that proximity to supermarkets selling healthier foods and increased walkability of a region predicted a lower BMI. Violent crime, often higher in low-income neighborhoods, has been associated with the development of obesity among young children, whereas a higher density of greenspace inversely correlated with obesity.[45]

Individual-Level Mechanisms

Individual-level factors include stigma, bias, and education and income. Stigma against individuals with obesity has multiple adverse ramifications on physical and psychological health. Although obesity has a complex cause that includes genetic and environmental factors, many mischaracterize obesity as a consequence of personal behavioral choices and blame individuals with obesity for their weight status.[8,46] In a phenomenon known as stereotype embodiment, individuals with obesity may internalize weight stigma.[47] This can lead to negative eating behaviors as a coping mechanism and worse mental and physical health outcomes.[48]

Weight stigma is also pervasive in medical practice, and existing literature has documented bias against individuals with obesity among primary care physicians, medical students, psychologists, and dentists.[46,49–52] In health-care settings, patients with higher BMI are more likely to have health problems misattributed to their weight status.[53] They are also falsely perceived as less adherent to medications.[54] These biases affect the provision of obesity care and health-care utilization. Indeed, patients with obesity who encounter weight stigma are less likely to access preventive care, adhere to treatment, and successfully lose weight.[46]

These stigmas are intimately tied to other mechanisms of obesity inequity. For example, a patient's SES, including their education, income, and occupation, affects their risk of developing obesity.[8] Individuals from lower socioeconomic backgrounds are more likely to have limited access to supermarkets or farmer's markets and instead may rely on convenience stores or fast food restaurants for their groceries.[55] Healthy foods may also be less affordable than processed or high-calorie food options.[55]

The impact of an individual's SES is also salient in accessing quality obesity care. Lifestyle intervention programs, a cornerstone of obesity treatment, are most successful when patients visit treatment facilities frequently and consistently.[56] However, disparities in transportation access and temporal constraints (eg, the restrictions imposed by working multiple jobs) may hamper a low-income patient's ability to adhere to treatment.[8] Previous studies have found that individuals who work more than 50 h/wk are more likely to have obesity, potentially due to limited opportunities for physical activity and restricted ability to access health-care services.[57]

It is crucial to note that these individual and structural mechanisms are often interconnected, creating a multiplicative effect on the development of obesity and exacerbating disparities in obesity prevalence and care.

CURRENT EFFORTS TO ADVANCE EQUITY

Owing to the current recognition that factors influencing the incidence of obesity and disparities in its treatment are intricate, multidisciplinary approaches targeting inequitable social structures, inequities in health system processes, and individual risky behaviors are essential for clinical and the clinical research that informs this care. In 2010, the National Institutes of Health established the National Institute of Minority Health and Disparities (NIMHD) to lead scientific research that improves minority health and reduces health disparities. The NIMHD has established a framework that accounts for various health determinants to inform our understanding of disparities in minority health and informs research funding at the NIH.[58]

Despite the explosion of research studies on addressing the obesity epidemic, a stark gap in implementation exists. Programs such as the National Diabetes Prevention Program (NDPP) have sought to address this gap. The NDPP is a public–private partnership started in 2010 that uses evidence-based, cost-effective interventions to tackle increasing rates of prediabetes and type 2 diabetes in the United States, emphasizing community-level interventions.[59] Through a lifestyle change program, community health workers are trained to provide evidence-based care to their communities. These efforts are supported by reevaluation of actions and evidence, such as the NIH workshop in 2017 to investigate and address socioeconomic factors that foster disparities in obesity and type 2 diabetes, as well as design culturally relevant and accessible prevention and treatment strategies.[15]

Digital health approaches also play an essential role in increasing access to obesity interventions. E-Health programs have shown evidence of short-term weight loss among ethnic minoritized individuals.[60] For example, a trial of an Internet-based program in low-income women on the supplemental nutrition assistance program (SNAP) produced more significant weight loss versus those on the SNAP program alone.[61] However, more studies are required to evaluate long-term effects and demonstrate clinically impactful results in this population.

Policy-level interventions also show promise in addressing equity in obesity prevention and management. Studies have shown that implementation of the SNAP program for women, infants, and children (WIC) in the low-income household was associated with declines in obesity prevalence for children enrolled between 2010 and 2016.[62] Another study found that The Healthy, Hunger-Free Kids Act of 2010 that improved nutrition standards through the National School Lunch Program had led to a significant reduction in obesity for children living in poverty each year after implementation, resulting in a 47% reduction in predicted obesity prevalence in 2018 had the legislation not been enacted. However, the legislation was not significantly associated with childhood obesity trends among general population overall.[63]

Finally, there is a paradigm shift in our framing of genetics or personal choice as explanations for disparities in obesity. Instead, it is increasingly recognized that discrimination, whether due to race, SES, or weight, is implicated in inequalities in the development and management of those with obesity.[64] There is also recognition that weight bias and stigma on the part of health-care providers affect the health-seeking practices of people with obesity.[65,66] However, significant gaps continue to exist in how this recognition can be translated to reducing bias. Furthermore, opportunities exist for reforming medical education and training to allow for more patient-centered care in patients with obesity.[67,68]

FUTURE DIRECTIONS

Efforts to improve health equity in obesity should consider the structural, community, and individual factors contributing to disparities in its prevalence. Social determinants of health, including health-care coverage and access, neighborhood, built environment, social context, education, and income, are upstream targets for intervention that could reduce disparities in obesity and its downstream effects. Obesity reduction efforts must work synergistically with a shared philosophy that equity is only reached through dismantling the pillars of social disadvantage to the full extent they are present.

At the policy level, the Affordable Care Act has been instrumental in improving health-care coverage among adults with obesity. However, baseline racial and ethnic disparities in coverage and access to care persist, such that non-Hispanic Black and Hispanic adults with obesity did not see improvements in access to care compared with White adults with obesity.[69] Further studies are needed to guide health policy-makers in determining the most effective means of ensuring the equitable distribution of health-care resources.

There is also a critical need for policy change that shifts insurance payor's framework of obesity. Glucagon-like peptide-1 receptor agonists have been approved for obesity by the FDA since 2014 yet remains covered by only 11% of marketplace plans.[70] Passage of legislation such as the Treat and Reduce Obesity Act in the United States would mobilize Medicare funding to increase access to medication and behavioral therapy.[71] Further, policy change can facilitate local obesity reduction efforts. These include financial incentives for the availability of perishable produce in small stores, beverage taxes, front-of-pack nutritional labeling, and restrictions on child-directed advertisement.[72,73]

Built environment characteristics such as high walk scores and street connectivity negatively correlate with obesity rates.[74] At the community level, interventions that optimize factors negatively associated with obesity in minoritized communities, such as public facilities, youth organizations, schools, and young men's christian association (YMCAs), may represent efficacious avenues for fundamentally promoting equity in obesity. Additional factors that might further decrease disparities include health-focused zoning code reform, funding of trails and paths, vacant lot renovation, urban forestry coordination, and increases in healthful food availability.[75]

From an individual standpoint, individualized risk assessment and improvement in patient–provider rapport and communication are essential to improving equity in obesity. Interventions focused on health behaviors rather than numerical weight have shown promise. The "Health at Every Size" (HAES) method has been suggested as an activity-based and nutrition-based approach impartial to a patient's numerical weight.[76] In 6 randomized controlled HAES trials, no adverse effects, including weight gain, were identified, and notable improvements in behavioral, psychological, clinical, and physiological outcomes.[77,78] Targeted physician bias education programs and the implementation of HAES primary care clinics in areas of high-obesity prevalence may reduce weight and identity stigma with cooperative effects due to their intrinsic intersectionality.

SUMMARY

Obesity is a complex, multifactorial chronic disease. Its increasing prevalence contributes to a host of other chronic illnesses, potentially decreased quality of life, and significant increases in the cost of health care. These adverse outcomes are disproportionately experienced by racial and ethnic minoritized communities and those of lower SES. Inequities in obesity and its negative effects are driven by systemic factors such as racial discrimination, neighborhood safety, access to healthy foods and quality health-care coverage, and individual-level factors such as weight stigma. Targeted research into the mechanisms behind disparities has helped elucidate them and contribute elements. However, further research is needed to guide the implementation of interventions that improve equity in obesity management and outcomes. Policy changes, such as expanded prescription coverage for obesity medication and changes in medical education and practice surrounding the management of obesity as a chronic disease, are further needed to improve health equity in obesity.

CLINICS CARE POINTS

- Obesity must be recognized as a chronic disease resulting from complex interactions between genetic, metabolic, behavioral, and environmental factors, and interventions to improve equity in obesity care must consider the variety of factors that contribute to its development.
- Similar to other chronic illnesses, health-care providers should be prepared to provide long-term management that consists of behavioral, medical, and possibly surgical interventions to reduce its burden and improve quality of life.
- Health-care providers must also recognize bias and stigma as barriers patients face in seeking care for managing obesity, should be aware of how they might contribute to discrimination and stigma, and be diligent in their language and actions so that they do not.
- Although BMI is a quick and widely used method to identify those with obesity, using it as a screening rather than a diagnostic tool may allow clinicians to better assess health risks at varying weight thresholds because it does not accurately capture weight due to lean muscle mass versus adiposity or differentiate visceral from subcutaneous adiposity, which may have implications in determining health risks based on weight.

DISCLOSURE

The authors declare that there is no conflict of interest associated with this article.

FUNDING

This project was supported by awards from the National Institutes of Health, United States NIDDK P30 DK040561 (F.C. Stanford) and U24 DK132733 (F.C. Stanford).

REFERENCES

1. Boutari C, Mantzoros CS. A 2022 update on the epidemiology of obesity and a call to action: as its twin COVID-19 pandemic appears to be receding, the obesity and dysmetabolism pandemic continues to rage on. Metabolism 2022;133: 155217.
2. Schwartz MW, Seeley RJ, Zeltser LM, et al. Obesity Pathogenesis: An Endocrine Society Scientific Statement. Endocr Rev 2017;38(4):267–96.
3. Bluher M. Adipose tissue dysfunction contributes to obesity related metabolic diseases. Best Pract Res Clin Endocrinol Metab 2013;27(2):163–77.
4. Taylor VH, Forhan M, Vigod SN, et al. The impact of obesity on quality of life. Best Pract Res Clin Endocrinol Metab 2013;27(2):139–46.
5. Kjellberg J, Tange Larsen A, Ibsen R, et al. The Socioeconomic Burden of Obesity. Obes Facts 2017;10(5):493–502.
6. Visscher TL, Seidell JC. The public health impact of obesity. Annu Rev Public Health 2001;22:355–75.
7. Hales CM, Carroll MD, Fryar CD, et al. Prevalence of Obesity and Severe Obesity Among Adults: United States, 2017-2018. NCHS Data Brief 2020;360:1–8.
8. Anekwe CV, Jarrell AR, Townsend MJ, et al. Socioeconomics of Obesity. Curr Obes Rep 2020;9(3):272–9.
9. Seidell JC, Halberstadt J. The global burden of obesity and the challenges of prevention. Ann Nutr Metab 2015;66(Suppl 2):7–12.

10. Pearce C, Rychetnik L, Wutzke S, et al. Obesity prevention and the role of hospital and community-based health services: a scoping review. BMC Health Serv Res 2019;19(1). https://doi.org/10.1186/s12913-019-4262-3.
11. Bray GA, Heisel WE, Afshin A, et al. The Science of Obesity Management: An Endocrine Society Scientific Statement. Endocr Rev 2018;39(2):79–132.
12. Kumanyika SK. A Framework for Increasing Equity Impact in Obesity Prevention. American Journal of Public Health 2019;109(10):1350–7.
13. Browne AJ, Varcoe CM, Wong ST, et al. Closing the health equity gap: evidence-based strategies for primary health care organizations. Int J Equity Health 2012; 11(1):59.
14. Ford-Gilboe M, Wathen CN, Varcoe C, et al. How Equity-Oriented Health Care Affects Health: Key Mechanisms and Implications for Primary Health Care Practice and Policy. Milbank Q 2018;96(4):635–71.
15. Thornton PL, Kumanyika SK, Gregg EW, et al. New research directions on disparities in obesity and type 2 diabetes. Ann N Y Acad Sci 2020;1461(1):5–24.
16. Fryar CD, Carroll MD, Afful J. Prevalence of overweight, obesity, and severe obesity among adults aged 20 and over: United States, 1960–1962 through 2017–2018. NCHS Health E-Stats 2020.
17. Wheeler SM, Bryant AS. Racial and Ethnic Disparities in Health and Health Care. Obstet Gynecol Clin North Am. Mar 2017;44(1):1–11.
18. Byrd AS, Toth AT, Stanford FC. Racial Disparities in Obesity Treatment. Curr Obes Rep 2018;7(2):130–8.
19. Cawley J, Rizzo JA. One pill makes you smaller: the demand for anti-obesity drugs. Adv Health Econ Health Serv Res 2007;17:149–83.
20. Mehta HB, Rajan SS, Aparasu RR, et al. Application of the nonlinear Blinder-Oaxaca decomposition to study racial/ethnic disparities in antiobesity medication use in the United States. Res Social Adm Pharm 2013;9(1):13–26.
21. Bomberg EM, Palzer EF, Rudser KD, et al. Anti-obesity medication prescriptions by race/ethnicity and use of an interpreter in a pediatric weight management clinic. Ther Adv Endocrinol Metab 2022;13. 20420188221090009.
22. Arterburn D, Westbrook EO, Terrell A. Weight control practices of severely obese patients who are not seeking bariatric surgery. Obesity 2013;21(8):1509–13.
23. Stephenson J. Report Finds Large Variation in States' Coverage for Obesity Treatments. JAMA Health Forum 2022;3(3):e220608.
24. Wee CC, Huskey KW, Bolcic-Jankovic D, et al. Sex, race, and consideration of bariatric surgery among primary care patients with moderate to severe obesity. J Gen Intern Med 2014;29(1):68–75.
25. Wallace AE, Young-Xu Y, Hartley D, et al. Racial, socioeconomic, and rural-urban disparities in obesity-related bariatric surgery. Obes Surg 2010;20(10):1354–60.
26. Bray GA, Frühbeck G, Ryan DH, et al. Management of obesity. Lancet 2016; 387(10031):1947–56.
27. Zhao J, Samaan JS, Abboud Y, et al. Racial disparities in bariatric surgery postoperative weight loss and co-morbidity resolution: a systematic review. Surg Obes Relat Dis 2021;17(10):1799–823.
28. Cossrow N, Falkner B. Race/ethnic issues in obesity and obesity-related comorbidities. J Clin Endocrinol Metab 2004;89(6):2590–4.
29. Ford ES, Giles WH, Dietz WH. Prevalence of the metabolic syndrome among US adults: findings from the third National Health and Nutrition Examination Survey. JAMA 2002;287(3):356–9.
30. Nuttall FQ. Body Mass Index: Obesity, BMI, and Health: A Critical Review. Nutr Today 2015;50(3):117–28.

31. Stanford FC, Lee M, Hur C. Race, Ethnicity, Sex, and Obesity: Is It Time to Personalize the Scale? Mayo Clin Proc 2019;94(2):362–3.
32. Taylor RW, Brooking L, Williams SM, et al. Body mass index and waist circumference cutoffs to define obesity in indigenous New Zealanders. Am J Clin Nutr 2010;92(2):390–7.
33. Examination Committee of Criteria for 'Obesity Disease' in Japan; Japan Society for the Study of Obesity. New criteria for 'obesity disease' in Japan. Circ J 2002; 66(11):987–92.
34. Shiwaku K, Anuurad E, Enkhmaa B, et al. Overweight Japanese with body mass indexes of 23.0-24.9 have higher risks for obesity-associated disorders: a comparison of Japanese and Mongolians. Int J Obes Relat Metab Disord 2004; 28(1):152–8.
35. Heymsfield SB, Peterson CM, Thomas DM, et al. Why are there race/ethnic differences in adult body mass index-adiposity relationships? A quantitative critical review. Obes Rev 2016;17(3):262–75.
36. Gaskin DJ, Dinwiddie GY, Chan KS, et al. Residential segregation and disparities in health care services utilization. Med Care Res Rev 2012;69(2):158–75.
37. Swope CB, Hernández D, Cushing LJ. The Relationship of Historical Redlining with Present-Day Neighborhood Environmental and Health Outcomes: A Scoping Review and Conceptual Model. J Urban Health 2022;99(6):959–83.
38. Shariff-Marco S, Klassen AC, Bowie JV. Racial/ethnic differences in self-reported racism and its association with cancer-related health behaviors. Am J Public Health 2010;100(2):364–74.
39. Butler C, Tull ES, Chambers EC, et al. Internalized racism, body fat distribution, and abnormal fasting glucose among African-Caribbean women in Dominica, West Indies. J Natl Med Assoc 2002;94(3):143–8.
40. Tull SE, Wickramasuriya T, Taylor J, et al. Relationship of internalized racism to abdominal obesity and blood pressure in Afro-Caribbean women. J Natl Med Assoc 1999;91(8):447–52.
41. Chambers EC, Tull ES, Fraser HS, et al. The relationship of internalized racism to body fat distribution and insulin resistance among African adolescent youth. J Natl Med Assoc 2004;96(12):1594–8.
42. Borrell LN, Graham L, Joseph SP. Associations of Neighborhood Safety and Neighborhood Support with Overweight and Obesity in US Children and Adolescents. Ethn Dis 2016;26(4):469–76.
43. Zick CD, Smith KR, Fan JX, et al. Running to the store? The relationship between neighborhood environments and the risk of obesity. Soc Sci Med 2009;69(10): 1493–500.
44. Rundle A, Neckerman KM, Freeman L, et al. Neighborhood food environment and walkability predict obesity in New York City. Environ Health Perspect 2009;117(3): 442–7.
45. Lovasi GS, Schwartz-Soicher O, Quinn JW, et al. Neighborhood safety and green space as predictors of obesity among preschool children from low-income families in New York City. Prev Med 2013;57(3):189–93.
46. Phelan SM, Burgess DJ, Yeazel MW, et al. Impact of weight bias and stigma on quality of care and outcomes for patients with obesity. Obes Rev 2015;16(4): 319–26.
47. Bajaj SS, Tu L, Stanford FC. Respectful language and putting the person first with obesity. Eur Heart J 2022;43(5):430.

48. Ratcliffe D, Ellison N. Obesity and internalized weight stigma: a formulation model for an emerging psychological problem. Behav Cogn Psychother 2015;43(2):239–52.
49. Miller DP Jr, Spangler JG, Vitolins MZ, et al. Are medical students aware of their anti obesity bias? Acad Med 2013;88(7):978–82.
50. Rubin R. Addressing Medicine's Bias Against Patients Who Are Overweight. JAMA 2019;321(10):925–7.
51. Tu L, Bajaj SS, Stanford FC. Locking ourselves into the past: the DentalSlim Diet Control device and an incomplete understanding of obesity. Int J Obes 2021;45(12):2513–4.
52. Tu L, Bajaj SS, Stanford FC. Promoting stigma. Br Dent J 2021;231(11):663–4.
53. Scott S, Currie J, Albert P, et al. Risk of misdiagnosis, health-related quality of life, and BMI in patients who are overweight with doctor-diagnosed asthma. Chest 2012;141(3):616–24.
54. Huizinga MM, Bleich SN, Beach MC, et al. Disparity in physician perception of patients' adherence to medications by obesity status. Obesity 2010;18(10):1932–7.
55. Rummo PE, Feldman JM, Lopez P, et al. Impact of Changes in the Food, Built, and Socioeconomic Environment on BMI in US Counties, BRFSS 2003-2012. Obesity 2020;28(1):31–9.
56. Webb VL, Wadden TA. Intensive Lifestyle Intervention for Obesity: Principles, Practices, and Results. Gastroenterology 2017;152(7):1752–64.
57. Park S, Pan L, Lankford T. Relationship between employment characteristics and obesity among employed U.S. adults. Am J Health Promot 2014;28(6):389–96.
58. Alvidrez J, Castille D, Laude-Sharp M, et al. The National Institute on Minority Health and Health Disparities Research Framework. Am J Public Health 2019;109(S1):S16–20.
59. Key National DPP Milestones | National Diabetes Prevention Program | Diabetes | CDC. Published December 27, 2022. Available at: https://www.cdc.gov/diabetes/prevention/milestones.htm. Accessed January 28, 2023.
60. Bennett GG, Steinberg DM, Stoute C, et al. Electronic health (eHealth) interventions for weight management among racial/ethnic minority adults: a systematic review. Obes Rev Off J Int Assoc Study Obes 2014;15(Suppl 4):146–58.
61. Phelan S, Hagobian T, Brannen A, et al. Effect of an Internet-Based Program on Weight Loss for Low-Income Postpartum Women. JAMA 2017;317(23):2381–91.
62. Pan L, Blanck HM, Park S, et al. State-Specific Prevalence of Obesity Among Children Aged 2-4 Years Enrolled in the Special Supplemental Nutrition Program for Women, Infants, and Children - United States, 2010-2016. MMWR Morb Mortal Wkly Rep 2019;68(46):1057–61.
63. Kenney EL, Barrett JL, Bleich SN, et al. Impact Of The Healthy, Hunger-Free Kids Act On Obesity Trends. Health Aff Proj Hope 2020;39(7):1122–9.
64. Duggan CP, Kurpad A, Stanford FC, et al. Race, ethnicity, and racism in the nutrition literature: an update for 2020. Am J Clin Nutr 2020;112(6):1409–14.
65. Tomiyama AJ, Carr D, Granberg EM, et al. How and why weight stigma drives the obesity 'epidemic' and harms health. BMC Med 2018;16:123.
66. Alberga AS, Edache IY, Forhan M, et al. Weight bias and health care utilization: a scoping review. Prim Health Care Res Dev 2019;20:e116.
67. Alberga AS, Pickering BJ, Alix Hayden K, et al. Weight bias reduction in health professionals: a systematic review. Clin Obes 2016;6(3):175–88.

68. Cardel MI, Newsome FA, Pearl RL, et al. Patient-Centered Care for Obesity: How Health Care Providers Can Treat Obesity While Actively Addressing Weight Stigma and Eating Disorder Risk. J Acad Nutr Diet 2022;122(6):1089–98.
69. Kendrick KN, Marcondes FO, Stanford FC, et al. Medicaid expansion and health care access for individuals with obesity in the United States. Obesity 2022;30(9): 1787–95.
70. Roser P, Bajaj SS, Stanford FC. International lack of equity in modern obesity therapy: the critical need for change in health policy. Int J Obes 2022;46(9):1571–2.
71. Text - S.596 - 117th Congress (2021-2022): Treat and Reduce Obesity Act of 2021. (2021, March 4). Available at: https://www.congress.gov/bill/117th-congress/senate-bill/596/text.
72. Lobstein T, Neveux M, Landon J. Costs, equity and acceptability of three policies to prevent obesity: A narrative review to support policy development. Obes Sci Pract 2020;6(5):562–83.
73. Blanck HM, Kim SA. Creating supportive nutrition environments for population health impact and health equity: an overview of the Nutrition and Obesity Policy Research and Evaluation Network's efforts. Am J Prev Med 2012;43(3 Suppl 2): S85–90.
74. Xu Y, Wang F. Built environment and obesity by urbanicity in the U.S. Health Place 2015;34:19–29.
75. Fedorowicz M, Schilling J, Bramhall E, et al. Leveraging the built environment for health equity. Washington, DC: Urban Institute; 2020.
76. Bombak A. Obesity, health at every size, and public health policy. Am J Public Health 2014;104(2):e60–7.
77. Bacon L, Aphramor L. Weight science: evaluating the evidence for a paradigm shift [published correction appears in Nutr J. Nutr J 2011;10:69.
78. Bacon L, Stern JS, Van Loan MD, et al. Size acceptance and intuitive eating improve health for obese, female chronic dieters. J Am Diet Assoc 2005; 105(6):929–36.

Racial and Ethnic Disparities in Metabolic Bone Disease

Lauren Y. Maldonado, MD, MPH[a,b,1], Linette Bosques, MD, PhD[a,1], Sara J. Cromer, MD[c], Sharl S. Azar, MD[d], Elaine W. Yu, MD, MMSc[c], Sherri-Ann M. Burnett-Bowie, MD, MPH[c,*]

KEYWORDS

• Metabolic bone disease • Osteoporosis • Metastatic bone disease
• Sickle cell disease • Health disparities

KEY POINTS

- Racial and ethnic disparities impact all aspects of medicine including bone health, particularly for patients with osteoporosis, metastatic cancer, and sickle cell disease.
- There are available screening tools and safe and effective therapies for osteoporosis; however, rates of screening and treatment are lower and disease morbidity is higher in minoritized populations. Fracture risk calculators and scoring mechanisms potentially worsen diagnostic and treatment disparities.
- Racial and ethnic minority groups disproportionately experience skeletal-related events due to metastatic bone disease yet experience greater delays in treatment and are more likely to present with significantly advanced disease.
- Metabolic bone disease significantly contributes to morbidity among patients with sickle cell disease, yet clinical guidelines to assist in timely screening and management do not exist.
- By providing clinical care points for bone disease, this review aims to close the margin on existing health care disparities and guide future research efforts.

Racial and ethnic disparities in care are pervasive and impact all aspects of medicine.[1] Here, we spotlight disparities in osteoporosis screening and treatment and in metastatic oncologic disease management. Furthermore, we discuss major unaddressed

[a] Department of Medicine, Massachusetts General Hospital and Harvard Medical School, 55 Fruit Street, Bigelow 730, Boston, MA 02114, USA; [b] Department of Pediatrics, MassGeneral Hospital for Children and Harvard Medical School, 175 Cambridge Street, Boston, MA 02114, USA; [c] Department of Medicine, Endocrine Division, Massachusetts General Hospital and Harvard Medical School, 50 Blossom Street, Thier 1051, Boston, MA 02114, USA; [d] Hematology and Medical Oncology Division, Department of Medicine, Massachusetts General Hospital and Harvard Medical School, 55 Fruit Street, Yawkey 9-536, Boston, MA 02114, USA
[1] Drs Maldonado and Bosques are co-first authors.
* Corresponding author.
E-mail address: sburnett-bowie@mgh.harvard.edu

Endocrinol Metab Clin N Am 52 (2023) 629–641
https://doi.org/10.1016/j.ecl.2023.05.004 endo.theclinics.com

gaps in bone health management in sickle cell disease (SCD). These diseases warrant focus because of the following.

- Osteoporosis, a leading cause of morbidity and mortality in the United States (US), is preventable and treatable.
- Cancer is either the first or second leading cause of death in all racial and ethnic groups in the US.[2,3]
- SCD, which affects 1 in 365 Black infants in the US, is associated with frailty, fractures, and significant chronic pain yet there is no consensus on bone health best practices.[4,5]

OSTEOPOROSIS

Introduction and Background

Osteoporosis is the most common metabolic bone disease (MBD) and is associated with significant comorbidity. More Asian, Black, Hispanic, and Native American women experience an osteoporosis-related fracture in 1 year than the combined number of those who experience breast cancer, myocardial infarction, and death related to chronic heart disease.[6] Screening is recommended for all women aged 65 years and older,[7,8] and some guidelines also recommend screening all men over 70 years.[7] Although safe and effective therapies exist to prevent osteoporosis-related morbidity and mortality, rates of screening[9] and treatment[10] in the general population are low, and racial and ethnic disparities exist at all stages of care.[11]

DISCUSSION

Health Disparities in Osteoporosis Diagnosis, Treatment, and Outcomes

Despite US recommendations for universal screening of women over 65 years of age, eligible Black women are less likely to be screened for osteoporosis than eligible White women, including after adjustment for possible mediating factors such as socioeconomic status, insurance, comorbidities, and health care utilization.[9,12–14] Similarly, among women who experience fragility hip fractures, both Black and Hispanic women are less likely to receive prior screening,[15] suggesting higher rates of preventable osteoporosis complications. Black women are also less likely to receive post-fracture bone dual-energy x-ray absorptiometry (DXA) screening.[14]

Among women who are diagnosed with osteoporosis, treatment disparities further exacerbate osteoporosis care inequities. Black women with osteoporosis are less likely to be prescribed calcium supplementation[16] and less likely to receive osteoporosis pharmacotherapy.[12,16,17] Although rates of screening, diagnosis, and treatment are lower among Black women, age-adjusted rates of fracture are also lower.[18,19] However, severe complications of fracture, including prolonged hospitalization, loss of mobility, and death, are higher among Black women.[20,21]

Osteoporosis screening, treatment, and complications data in men and women of Hispanic, East Asian, South Asian, Native American (American Indian or First Nations), or other race and ethnicity are less established than that among Black and White individuals. Bone mineral density (BMD) and fracture risk for Hispanic women usually fall between that of Black and White women. Among Asian women, BMD is lower but fracture risk is also lower than Black and White women.[18,22–25] Fracture rates among Native American and South Asian women are high and generally comparable to White women.[18,26] Native American persons may have elevated mortality following fracture, as seen among Black individuals.[27] Regarding treatment risks, East Asian women have greater risk than White women of atypical femoral fracture and osteonecrosis of the jaw when treated with bisphosphonates.[28,29] Increased attention to these populations is warranted to fully understand the impact of osteoporosis in diverse women.

Systems-Level Factors Impacting Racial and Ethnic Differences in Osteoporosis Care

To address disparities in osteoporosis, we must understand how our medical practices contribute to them. First, BMD is lower[23–25] and rates of osteoporosis and fracture are higher[18,19] among White women than among Black or Hispanic women, whereas Asian women have lower BMD[22] but also lower rates of fracture[18] than White women. Because of this, race and ethnicity have been used as factors in the Fracture Risk Assessment Tool (FRAX), a commonly used clinical risk score that guides osteoporosis therapy recommendations.[30] This practice is currently under review as it may exacerbate osteoporosis treatment disparities; furthermore, as populations become more heterogeneous, it will be increasingly challenging to classify individuals using these categories (eg, how should FRAX be applied to someone with Asian and Black parents). Similarly, DXA interpretation in women of non-White race and ethnicity is complicated because many labs generate T-scores by comparing to White reference databases. In certain racial and ethnic groups, this practice may falsely elevate T-scores and potentially underestimate fracture risk. Finally, awareness of population-level differences in BMD and fracture risk may negatively impact providers' decisions to refer a patient for screening DXA, despite recommendations for universal DXA screening of women over age 65 years and the fact that complication rates after fracture are higher among Black women.[20,21] Safe and effective therapies, like alendronate and zoledronic acid, exist to treat osteoporosis; however, many patients go without treatment due to inequities in screening or treatment.[31] Thus, it is critical to correct these systems-level factors, which exacerbate disparities, to ensure equitable fracture prevention measures. Please see the *Clinics Care Points* for clinical recommendations.

SKELETAL METASTASES IN CANCER

Introduction and Background

Cancer is a leading cause of death in all racial and ethnic groups in the US.[2,3] In 2019, there were 415,083 new cancer cases and 136,422 cancer deaths among non-White individuals.[32] More than 90% of cancer-related deaths are caused by metastasis.[33] Bone is among the most common site of metastasis for malignancies originating in the breast, prostate, thyroid, lung, and kidney.[34–36] Skeletal-related events (SREs), including bone pain, pathologic fractures, spinal cord compression, bone marrow infiltration, and hypercalcemia, reduce overall survival and are associated with loss of social functioning, decreased quality of life, and significant medical cost.[35] Racial and ethnic disparities in the incidence and outcome of cancers originating in bone also exist. Black patients are twice as likely to develop multiple myeloma and experience worse outcomes following diagnosis as compared to non-Hispanic White patients.[37,38] To raise awareness and guide future research efforts, this review aims to highlight racial and ethnic disparities in the incidence and management of metastatic bone disease (MtBD).

DISCUSSION

Racial, Ethnic, and Socioeconomic Differences in the Incidence of Metastatic Bone Disease

The Surveillance, Epidemiology, and Ends Results database identified a higher incidence of MtBD from lung, prostate, and breast cancer in non-Hispanic Black patients compared to non-Hispanic White, Native American, Alaskan Native, Asian Pacific

Islander, and Hispanic patients.[39] Notably, lower socioeconomic status is an independent risk factor for worse disease specific survival for patients with MtBD associated with lung, prostate, breast, and colon cancer.[40] Similarly, a retrospective study of 35,808 women diagnosed with stage I–III breast cancer found that Black women are 60% more likely than White women to develop metastases (17% vs. 10%, respectively),[41] with the most common metastasis site being bone (~42%). Another study of ~ 520,000 patients with breast, prostate, or colorectal cancer revealed that a significantly higher proportion of non-Hispanic Black (11%) and Hispanic (10%) patients present with *de novo* metastasis when compared to non-Hispanic White (9%) patients ($P < 0.001$).[42] Furthermore, non-Hispanic Black patients have 50% higher hazards for mortality when compared to non-Hispanic White patients (hazard ratio [HR]: 1.50, 95% confidence interval [CI]: 1.43–1.58).

Racial and ethnic differences in SREs exist among patients with breast cancer-associated MtBD.[43] Native American patients have the highest rate of SRE prior to bisphosphonate therapy at ~ 67% compared to non-Hispanic White (63%) and Hispanic (36%) patients.[43] Within 1 year of initiating treatment, 39% of Native American patients develop an SRE compared to 21% and 8% of Hispanic and non-Hispanic White patients, respectively.[43] Among elderly men with metastatic prostate cancer, White patients are 27% more likely to develop SREs compared with Black patients.[44] However, Black patients incur higher health care utilization costs for the treatment of SREs, with bone surgery being the most expensive component.[44]

Disparities in the Management and Consequences of Metastatic Bone Disease

Management of MtBD involves maximizing analgesia, preserving physical function, and minimizing SREs using medications, radiation therapy, and, in some cases, surgery.[35] Bisphosphonates and denosumab can be used to further reduce the risk of SREs.[45] Racial and ethnic disparities, however, even exist in the initiation of bisphosphonate therapy for multiple myeloma, with White patients being more likely and Black patients less likely to receive IV bisphosphonate treatment, despite multiple myeloma being more prevalent in Black individuals.[37,38,46]

Disparities in clinical outcomes of patients with MtBD also exist. In a retrospective analysis of 145,000 patients (including ~ 75% White, 14% Black, 8% Hispanic, and 3% Asian patients) admitted with skeletal metastases, Asian, Black, and Hispanic patients had poorer outcomes than White patients.[47] Although 80% to 95% of patients with metastatic spine disease present with back pain,[48] Black patients are significantly more likely to present with advanced symptoms, including spinal cord compression.[47] Lower cancer screening rates and delayed diagnoses contribute to these advanced cancer presentations in vulnerable populations.[49,50] Furthermore, poor neurologic outcomes occur in patients presenting with 48 hours or more of spinal cord compression.[51,52] Thus, early detection is key for favorable outcomes. Together with Hispanic patients, Black patients also have higher rates of paralysis.[47] Concerningly, racial disparities exist in the management of spinal cord compression,[47] which is usually managed with surgery and radiation treatment.[51,52] Black patients are less likely to undergo surgical intervention (OR 0.71; 95% CI, 0.62–0.82), and significantly more likely to experience an in-hospital complication (OR 1.25; 95% CI, 1.12–1.40).[47] Please see the *Clinics Care Points* for clinical recommendations.

METABOLIC BONE DISEASE IN SICKLE CELL DISEASE

Introduction and Background

SCD disproportionately affects Black and Hispanic populations.[4] Among the 100,000 individuals living with SCD in the US, 90% are Black, 9% are Hispanic, and 1% are

Middle Eastern, Indian, or other descent.[53] Much of SCD's long-term morbidity is due to associated MBD; however, complications can be challenging to diagnose, particularly in patients with chronic pain. Despite SCD's prevalence and complexity, screening tools to identify and guidelines to care for patients at highest risk of developing MBD do not yet exist. In the US, structural systemic injustices and racism experienced by minoritized populations perpetuate disparate outcomes.[54]

SCD predominantly impacts bone via ischemia. Affected hemoglobin may sickle in low-oxygen environments, leading to venous and end-arterial thromboses, tissue hypoxia, and necrosis. When bone ischemia occurs, vaso-occlusive bone pain, osteonecrosis, or infection (eg, osteomyelitis, septic arthritis) may develop. Chronic hemolysis increases risk for marrow hyperplasia and bony deformities.[55] These complications can cause severe pain, and lead to chronic immobility and/or decreased quality of life. Patients with SCD have an elevated risk of developing osteoporosis and fractures due to comorbid conditions (eg, low body weight, higher incidence of tobacco use, malnutrition, hypogonadism).[56] Further, there are significant racial disparities in SCD-related complications, namely Black patients are more likely to experience sickle cell crises and blindness as compared to White patients.[57]

Altogether, these conditions contribute to the significantly decreased life expectancy in patients with SCD.[58] The average lifespan for a patient living with SCD is 20 years shorter than the average population and most patients will not achieve their 45th birthday.[59] Furthermore, SCD produces chronic changes on the cellular, organ, and physical levels that mimic syndromes of accelerated aging.[60] These sobering data underscore the urgent need for early bone disease screening among patients with SCD to ensure relevant and timely impact.

DISCUSSION

Avascular Necrosis

Avascular necrosis (AVN) is one of the most common bone-related SCD complications. AVN occurs when blood supply to long bone epiphyses at weight-bearing joints is occluded, leading to microfractures, trabecular bone collapse, and articular surface collapse. In SCD, AVN often first presents in childhood, with 28% of patients experiencing femoral head AVN[61]; prevalence increases to ~ 50% in adulthood, with 77% of adults progressing to joint collapse.[62,63] Risk for developing AVN is higher in patients with Hemoglobin SS and Hemoglobin SC subtypes and increases with age (particularly above 30 years).[63–65] Conversely, patients with increased hemoglobin F are less likely to have AVN.[66] Other risk factors for AVN include male sex, high body mass index (BMI), low BMD, recurrent vaso-occlusive pain, and prior diagnosis of acute chest syndrome.[64]

AVN is often asymptomatic and incidentally found on imaging, complicating timely diagnosis. Among symptomatic patients, AVN most commonly affects the humeral head, femoral head, and patellar surface, with bilateral and multiple joint involvement being possible.[63] Referred pain to the back, buttocks, groin or knee and decreased range of motion or antalgic gait should prompt consideration. Scoring systems integrate physical and radiographic findings to risk stratify patients and assist diagnosis; unfortunately, there are no validated diagnostic biomarkers.[67,68] Given these limitations, clinicians should have a low threshold to obtain imaging in patients with SCD for whom AVN is suspected and consider universal screening (eg, with MRI though no current expert consensus exists) for patients with SCD before the age of 30 years to assist in early detection.

Despite the disproportionate incidence of AVN in SCD, clinical trial data regarding AVN treatment are sparse. AVN is typically managed nonsurgically with analgesia, hydration, non-weight bearing, and physical therapy.[69] Escalation to surgical core decompression, tissue grafting, and/or arthroplasty typically follows failed conservative management; however, data do not strongly support long-term improvement in clinical outcomes.[70,71] New therapies, including autologous bone marrow-derived stem cell injections, demonstrate promise for slowing disease progression, though long-term outcomes data are limited and broad dissemination may be cost-prohibited.[70] With the availability of newer orthopedic interventions that could potentially delay or prevent total joint replacement, the need for earlier AVN detection is that much more underscored.

Few randomized controlled trials have investigated if bisphosphonates slow or prevent early femoral head collapse in AVN, and most studies have included non-SCD etiologies of AVN (eg, glucocorticoids, systemic lupus, idiopathic). Data are discordant regarding alendronate, with one study demonstrating significant associations between alendronate use and reduction in collapse at 2 years and another finding no significant associations between use and disease reduction, progression to arthroplasty, or improvement in quality of life among a similar cohort (AVN stage II or III).[72,73] Similarly, in an open-label randomized trial, zoledronic acid did not significantly reduce prevention of collapse or progression to arthroplasty at 2 years.[74] There is limited non-randomized comparative data demonstrating greater efficacy of teriparatide in reducing the rate of advanced collapse versus alendronate.[75]

There is limited, non-placebo-controlled data supporting the use of IV bisphosphonates for analgesia among children with SCD-related AVN. In 23 children with SCD, IV bisphosphonates improved or resolved AVN-associated bone pain without triggering complications (eg, hemolysis, painful vaso-occlusive events, stroke) or developing therapy-related complications (eg, osteonecrosis of the jaw).[76] After ensuring normal serum calcium and 25-hydroxyvitamin D (25OHD), patients were treated with IV pamidronate, IV zoledronic acid, or pamidronate followed by zoledronic acid. Analgesia was noted within 1 to 6 months and continued through 1.5 years without significant pain recurrence. Clinical questions remain, including alternative indications for bisphosphonates and long-term safety (however, in pediatric patients with osteogenesis imperfecta and adult patients with low BMD, bisphosphonates are shown to be safe).[31,77]

Bone Mineral Density and Vitamin D

Approximately, 72% of young adults with SCD (mean age 34 years) have low BMD; in comparison, ~ 44% of adults 50 years of age or older have low BMD based on National Health and Nutrition Examination Survey (NHANES) data.[78,79] Mechanisms leading to BMD loss in SCD are multifactorial and hypothesized to include vitamin D deficiency, marrow expansion due to chronic hemolysis and compensatory erythropoiesis, iron overload, vaso-occlusion-associated ischemia, and an imbalance between osteoblasts and osteoclasts due to tissue hypoxia and erythropoietin release.[80] Disease management should emphasize early detection and prevention.

Low vitamin D (insufficiency 25OHD < 20 ng/mL; deficiency < 12 ng/mL) is a preventable risk factor for developing low BMD.[81] In NHANES, ~5% of individuals 1 year of age or older had 25OHD less than 12 ng/mL and 18% 25OHD between 12 to 19 ng/mL.[82] Notably, ~ 82% of Black and 69% of Hispanic individuals have 25OHD less than 20 ng/mL[83]; comparatively, the reported prevalence of 25OHD less than 20 ng'/mL among pediatric and adult SCD patients ranges from ~ 56 to 96%.[84] Among studies with comparison groups, patients with SCD have higher prevalence of suboptimal vitamin D levels versus matched non-SCD controls. Notably, in pediatric studies of severe deficiency (25OHD < 11 ng/mL) where patients with homozygous SS disease were compared to matched controls, one study reported greater prevalence of severe deficiency in those with Hemoglobin SS (65%) versus healthy Black adults (6%) or Black children (0%).[85,86] The other study similarly found that adjusted for season and age, those with SCD were 5.3 (95% CI: 2.5, 8.2) times more likely to be vitamin D deficient than healthy controls.[85,86]

Individuals with SCD may be more susceptible to low vitamin D levels because of physiologic (eg, increased metabolism due to high cell turnover, decreased synthesis from sunlight due to increased skin pigmentation, decreased appetite and intestinal absorption in SCD, renal impairment) and structural factors (eg, limited access to nutritious, vitamin D rich foods).[84] Although the USPSTF 2021 recommendations state that there is insubstantial evidence to support routinely screening asymptomatic adults for vitamin D deficiency, these recommendations do not provide clear guidance on screening patients at increased risk for low vitamin D.[87] Recent reviews also suggest insufficient evidence to support empiric repletion in SCD.[88] However, given the disproportionate prevalence of deficiency and comorbidity if untreated, clinicians should consider empirically initiating vitamin D supplementation in all SCD patients, and measuring parathyroid hormone (PTH) and serum 25OHD annually.

Fragility Fractures and Role for Bisphosphonates in Low Bone Mineral Density

Among SCD patients with low BMD, having 25OHD less than 12 ng/mL, low BMI, elevated PTH, C-terminal telopeptides of type 1 collagen, and bone-specific alkaline phosphatase increases fracture risk.[89] In a mostly female cohort of 71 patients with SCD, with $\sim$ 15% of patients having osteoporosis based on T-score, serum lactate dehydrogenase (LDH) and aspartate aminotransferase (AST) (not BMD) predicted vertebral fracture severity.[90] The mechanism by which LDH or AST was associated with increased fracture risk is unknown, though elevations in LDH may reflect more hemolytic SCD phenotypes. Additional studies are needed to understand the role LDH and liver function screening may play in predicting bone health in SCD.

There are limited data on bisphosphonate therapy in patients with both SCD and low BMD. Additional studies should evaluate the role of bisphosphonates in the treatment of osteoporosis in patients with SCD. Please see the *Clinics Care Points* for clinical recommendations.

SUMMARY

Racial and ethnic health disparities in screening and treatment of osteoporosis, MtBD, and SCD are pervasive. Highlighting these disparities and underscoring gaps in understanding sheds light on important areas for future research. Further studies should clarify the impact of these diseases on minoritized populations and solidify recommendations for treatment and management.

CLINICS CARE POINTS

Osteoporosis:

- Screen all women aged over 65 years and all men aged over 70 for osteoporosis, regardless of race and ethnicity. People with increased risk of fracture (eg, secondary to early menopause, steroid use, SCD) should be screened earlier.
- All individuals with bone dual energy x-ray absorptiometry (DXA)-defined osteoporosis (T-score ≤ -2.5) or a fragility fracture of the spine, hip, wrist, humerus, pelvis, or ribs should be treated for osteoporosis. Currently, fewer than 10% of women with osteoporosis receive effective therapy in a timely manner.

- Bisphosphonates, such as alendronate and zoledronic acid, are first-line therapy for osteoporosis. Although bisphosphonates can have serious side effects, these are very rare, and the overall safety profile of bisphosphonates is very good.
- Current practices, including use of race and ethnicity in fracture risk calculation and use of a White reference database when calculating T-scores, may contribute to racial and ethnic disparities.
- Further studies that examine how best to close gaps in care are urgently needed to improve both overall osteoporosis care and address significant disparities in achieving guideline-concordant care.

Skeletal metastases in cancer:

- Racial and ethnic minoritized populations are at higher risk of developing SREs, are less likely to be appropriately treated for SREs, and have worse outcomes from MtBD.
- Patients at high risk of MtBD should be advised to seek immediate medical care if they develop new onset back pain or neurologic symptoms.
- Bisphosphonates or denosumab should be used to minimize the risk of SREs in patients with MtBD.
- Spine imaging should be obtained in patients with suspected spinal metastases.
- Definitive treatment should be started within 24 hours of a confirmed diagnosis of spinal cord compression.

Metabolic bone disease in SCD:

- Black and Hispanic populations are disproportionately affected by SCD and are unlikely to live past age 45 years; as such, there is an urgent need for early and timely bone disease screening.
- People with SCD are at elevated risk of AVN leading to short- and long-term morbidity. As AVN may be asymptomatic, clinicians should obtain radiographs in patients with new joint symptoms or gait instability.
- Clinicians should consider universally screening individuals with SCD for AVN prior to age 30 years given the likelihood of asymptomatic disease and possibility of early intervention to slow progression.
- Vitamin D deficiency is highly prevalent among individuals with SCD. We recommend daily intake of at least 2000 units of cholecalciferol or ergocalciferol and ~ 1000 mg of calcium.
- Black patients with SCD have higher rates of osteopenia/osteoporosis than Black individuals without SCD. Studies are needed to understand when patients with SCD should be screened with DXA.
- Routine guidelines for treating low BMD should be implemented in patients with SCD, and additional research specific to the treatment of AVN and metabolic bone disease in SCD populations is necessary.

DISCLOSURE

S.J. Cromer reports a close family member employed by a Johnson & Johnson company. S.S. Azar has received grant support from Global Blood Therapeutics and Vertex Pharmaceuticals, United States. E.W. Yu has received grant support from Amgen, Inc, United States. S.M. Burnett-Bowie is a member of the clinical advisory board for Upliv Health. Other authors do not have any relevant financial disclosures.

REFERENCES

1. Institute of Medicine (US). Committee on understanding and eliminating racial and ethnic disparities in health care. In: Smedley BD, Stith AY, Nelson AR, editors. Unequal treatment: confronting racial and ethnic disparities in health care. Washington, DC: National Academies Press (US) Copyright; 2002. by the National Academy of Sciences. All rights reserved 2003.

2. Centers for Disease Control and Prevention. Leading Causes of Death in Females, United States. https://www.cdc.gov/women/lcod/index.htm.
3. Centers for Disease Control and Prevention. Leading Causes of Death in Males, United States. https://www.cdc.gov/minorityhealth/lcod/index.htm.
4. Centers for Disease Control and Prevention. Data and Statistics on Sickle Cell Disease. https://www.cdc.gov/ncbddd/sicklecell/data.html#print.
5. Bryson S. UConn Team Awarded Nearly $3M to Study Bone Loss in Sickle Cell. 2023. https://sicklecellanemianews.com/news/bone-loss-scd-focus-nearly-3m-awarded-uconn-scientists/.
6. Cauley JA, Wampler NS, Barnhart JM, et al. Incidence of fractures compared to cardiovascular disease and breast cancer: the Women's Health Initiative Observational Study. Osteoporos Int 2008;19(12):1717–23.
7. Cosman F, Beur SJd, LeBoff MS, et al. Clinician's Guide to Prevention and Treatment of Osteoporosis. Osteoporosis International 2014;25(10):2359.
8. US Preventive Services Task Force. Screening for Osteoporosis to Prevent Fractures: US Preventive Services Task Force Recommendation Statement. JAMA 2018;319(24):2521–31.
9. Gillespie CW, Morin PE. Trends and Disparities in Osteoporosis Screening Among Women in the United States, 2008-2014. Am J Med 2017;130(3):306–16.
10. Cromer SJ, D'Silva KM, Yu EW, et al. Secular Trends in the Pharmacologic Treatment of Osteoporosis and Malignancy-Related Bone Disease from 2009 to 2020. J Gen Intern Med 2022;37(8):1917–24.
11. Ruiz-Esteves KN, Teysir J, Schatoff D, et al. Disparities in osteoporosis care among postmenopausal women in the United States. Maturitas 2022;156:25–9.
12. Hamrick I, Cao Q, Agbafe-Mosley D, et al. Osteoporosis Healthcare Disparities in Postmenopausal Women. J Wom Health 2012;21(12):1232–6.
13. Miller RG, Ashar BH, Cohen J, et al. Disparities in osteoporosis screening between at-risk African-American and white women. J Gen Intern Med 2005; 20(9):847–51.
14. Mudano AS, Casebeer L, Patino F, et al. Racial disparities in osteoporosis prevention in a managed care population. South Med J 2003;96(5):445–51.
15. Neuner JM, Zhang X, Sparapani R, et al. Racial and Socioeconomic Disparities in Bone Density Testing Before and After Hip Fracture. J Gen Intern Med 2007; 22(9):1239–45.
16. Wei GS, Jackson JL, Herbers JE. Ethnic disparity in the treatment of women with established low bone mass. J Am Med Wom Assoc 2003;58(3):173–7.
17. Cunningham TD, Di Pace BS, Ullal J. Osteoporosis treatment disparities: a 6-year aggregate analysis from national survey data. Osteoporosis International 2014; 25(9):2199–208.
18. Cauley JA, Wu L, Wampler NS, et al. Clinical Risk Factors for Fractures in Multi-Ethnic Women: The Women's Health Initiative. J Bone Miner Res 2007;22(11): 1816–26.
19. Tsai AJ. Disparities in osteoporosis by race/ethnicity, education, work status, immigrant status, and economic status in the United States. Eur J Intern Med 2019;64:85–9.
20. Kellie SE, Brody JA. Sex-specific and race-specific hip fracture rates. Am J Publ Health 1990;80(3):326–8.
21. Penrod JD, Litke A, Hawkes WG, et al. The Association of Race, Gender, and Comorbidity With Mortality and Function After Hip Fracture. The journals of gerontology Series A, Biological sciences and medical sciences 2008;63(8):867–72.

22. Lo JC, Chandra M, Lee C, et al. Bone Mineral Density in Older U.S. Filipino, Chinese, Japanese, and White Women. J Am Geriatr Soc 2020;68(11):2656–61.
23. Looker AC, Melton LJ, Borrud LG, et al. Lumbar spine bone mineral density in US adults: demographic patterns and relationship with femur neck skeletal status. Osteoporos Int 2012;23(4):1351–60.
24. Looker AC, Melton LJ, Harris TB, et al. Prevalence and Trends in Low Femur Bone Density Among Older US Adults: NHANES 2005–2006 Compared With NHANES III. J Bone Miner Res 2010;25(1):64–71.
25. Xu Y, Wu Q. Decreasing Trend of Bone Mineral Density in US Multiethnic Population: Analysis of Continuous NHANES 2005 - 2014. Osteoporos Int 2018;29(11): 2437–46.
26. Khandewal S, Chandra M, Lo JC. Clinical characteristics, bone mineral density and non-vertebral osteoporotic fracture outcomes among post-menopausal U.S. South Asian Women. Bone 2012;51(6):1025–8.
27. Leslie WD, Brennan SL, Prior HJ, et al. The contributions of First Nations ethnicity, income, and delays in surgery on mortality post-fracture: a population-based analysis. Osteoporosis International 2013;24(4):1247–56.
28. Lo JC, Hui RL, Grimsrud CD, et al. The Association of Race/Ethnicity and Risk of Atypical Femur Fracture among Older Women Receiving Oral Bisphosphonate Therapy. Bone 2016;85:142.
29. Taguchi A, Shiraki M, Morrison A, et al. Antiresorptive agent-related osteonecrosis of the jaw in osteoporosis patients from Asian countries. Osteoporosis and Sarcopenia 2017;3(2):64–74.
30. Kanis JA, Johnell O, Oden A, et al. FRAX™ and the assessment of fracture probability in men and women from the UK. Osteoporosis International 2008;19(4): 385–97.
31. Reid IR, Horne AM, Mihov B, et al. Fracture Prevention with Zoledronate in Older Women with Osteopenia. N Engl J Med 2018;379(25):2407–16.
32. U.S. Cancer Statistics Working Group. U.S. Cancer statistics data visualizations tool, based on 2021 submission data (1999-2019). Washington, DC: U.S. Department of Health and Human Services, Centers for Disease Control and Prevention and National Cancer Institute; 2019.
33. Ganesh K, Massague J. Targeting metastatic cancer. Nat Med 2021;27(1):34–44.
34. Coleman RE. Skeletal complications of malignancy. Cancer 1997;80(8 Suppl): 1588–94.
35. Coleman RE, Croucher PI, Padhani AR, et al. Bone metastases. Nat Rev Dis Primers 2020;6(1):83.
36. Wang M, Xia F, Wei Y, et al. Molecular mechanisms and clinical management of cancer bone metastasis. Bone Res 2020;8(1):30.
37. Sun T, Wang S, Sun H, et al. Improved survival in multiple myeloma, with a diminishing racial gap and a widening socioeconomic status gap over three decades. Leuk Lymphoma 2018;59(1):49–58.
38. Brown LM, Gridley G, Check D, et al. Risk of multiple myeloma and monoclonal gammopathy of undetermined significance among white and black male United States veterans with prior autoimmune, infectious, inflammatory, and allergic disorders. Blood 2008;111(7):3388–94.
39. Jawad MU, Pollock BH, Wise BL, et al. Sex, racial/ethnic and socioeconomic disparities in patients with metastatic bone disease. J Surg Oncol 2022;125(4): 766–74.

40. Jawad MU, Pollock BH, Wise BL, et al. Socioeconomic and insurance-related disparities in disease-specific survival among patients with metastatic bone disease. J Surg Oncol 2023;127(1):159–73.
41. Schootman M, Jeffe DB, Gillanders WE, et al. Racial disparities in the development of breast cancer metastases among older women: a multilevel study. Cancer 2009;115(4):731–40.
42. Akinyemiju T, Sakhuja S, Waterbor J, et al. Racial/ethnic disparities in de novo metastases sites and survival outcomes for patients with primary breast, colorectal, and prostate cancer. Cancer Med 2018;7(4):1183–93.
43. Zheng Z, Chen L, Lee JH, et al. Racial/ethnic disparities in skeletal-related events among women treated with bisphosphonate therapy for bone metastasis secondary to breast cancer. Clin Oncol, 2018, 36(15_suppl), e13092-e13092.
44. Jayasekera J, Onukwugha E, Bikov K, et al. Racial variation in the clinical and economic burden of skeletal-related events among elderly men with stage IV metastatic prostate cancer. Expert Rev Pharmacoecon Outcomes Res 2015; 15(3):471–85.
45. Saylor PJ, Rumble RB, Tagawa S, et al. Bone Health and Bone-Targeted Therapies for Prostate Cancer: ASCO Endorsement of a Cancer Care Ontario Guideline. J Clin Oncol 2020;38(15):1736–43.
46. Zhou J, Sweiss K, Nutescu EA, et al. Racial Disparities in Intravenous Bisphosphonate Use Among Older Patients With Multiple Myeloma Enrolled in Medicare. JCO Oncol Pract 2021;17(3):e294–312.
47. De la Garza Ramos R, Benton JA, Gelfand Y, et al. Racial disparities in clinical presentation, type of intervention, and in-hospital outcomes of patients with metastatic spine disease: An analysis of 145,809 admissions in the United States. Cancer Epidemiol 2020;68:101792.
48. Bach F, Larsen BH, Rohde K, et al. Metastatic spinal cord compression. Occurrence, symptoms, clinical presentations and prognosis in 398 patients with spinal cord compression. Acta Neurochir 1990;107(1–2):37–43.
49. Virnig BA, Baxter NN, Habermann EB, et al. A matter of race: early-versus late-stage cancer diagnosis. Health Aff 2009;28(1):160–8.
50. Seeff LC, Nadel MR, Klabunde CN, et al. Patterns and predictors of colorectal cancer test use in the adult U.S. population. Cancer 2004;100(10):2093–103.
51. Laufer I, Zuckerman SL, Bird JE, et al. Predicting Neurologic Recovery after Surgery in Patients with Deficits Secondary to MESCC: Systematic Review. Spine 2016;41(Suppl 20):S224–30.
52. Singleton JM, Hefner M. Spinal cord compression. Treasure Island, FL: StatPearls; 2022.
53. Brousseau DC, Panepinto JA, Nimmer M, et al. The number of people with sickle-cell disease in the United States: national and state estimates. Am J Hematol 2010;85(1):77–8.
54. Lee L, Smith-Whitley K, Banks S, et al. Reducing Health Care Disparities in Sickle Cell Disease: A Review. Public Health Rep 2019;134(6):599–607.
55. Almeida A, Roberts I. Bone involvement in sickle cell disease. Br J Haematol 2005;129(4):482–90.
56. Cummings SR, Nevitt MC, Browner WS, et al. Risk factors for hip fracture in white women. Study of Osteoporotic Fractures Research Group. N Engl J Med 1995; 332(12):767–73.
57. Pokhrel A, Olayemi A, Ogbonda S, et al. Racial and ethnic differences in sickle cell disease within the United States: From demographics to outcomes. Eur J Haematol 2023. https://doi.org/10.1111/ejh.13936.

58. Lin K, Barton MBUS. Preventive Services Task Force Evidence Syntheses, formerly Systematic Evidence Reviews. Screening for hemoglobinopathies in newborns: reaffirmation update for the US preventive services task force. Agency for Healthcare Research and Quality (US); 2007.
59. Kavanagh PL, Fasipe TA, Wun T. Sickle Cell Disease: A Review. JAMA 2022; 328(1):57–68.
60. Idris IM, Botchwey EA, Hyacinth HI. Sickle cell disease as an accelerated aging syndrome. Exp Biol Med (Maywood) 2022;247(4):368–74.
61. Adekile AD, Gupta R, Al-Khayat A, et al. Risk of avascular necrosis of the femoral head in children with sickle cell disease on hydroxyurea: MRI evaluation. Pediatr Blood Cancer 2019;66(2):e27503.
62. Hernigou P, Habibi A, Bachir D, et al. The natural history of asymptomatic osteonecrosis of the femoral head in adults with sickle cell disease. J Bone Joint Surg 2006;88(12):2565–72.
63. Milner PF, Kraus AP, Sebes JI, et al. Sickle cell disease as a cause of osteonecrosis of the femoral head. N Engl J Med 1991;325(21):1476–81.
64. Adesina OO, Neumayr LD. Osteonecrosis in sickle cell disease: an update on risk factors, diagnosis, and management. Hematology Am Soc Hematol Educ Program 2019;2019(1):351–8.
65. Powars DR, Chan LS, Hiti A, et al. Outcome of sickle cell anemia: a 4-decade observational study of 1056 patients. Medicine (Baltim) 2005;84(6):363–76.
66. Hawker H, Neilson H, Hayes RJ, et al. Haematological factors associated with avascular necrosis of the femoral head in homozygous sickle cell disease. Br J Haematol 1982;50(1):29–34.
67. Aguilar CM, Neumayr LD, Eggleston BE, et al. Clinical evaluation of avascular necrosis in patients with sickle cell disease: Children's Hospital Oakland Hip Evaluation Scale–a modification of the Harris Hip Score. Arch Phys Med Rehabil 2005;86(7):1369–75.
68. University of Pennsylvannia. The University of Pennsylvania Classification of Osteonecrosis. https://radiologykey.com/the-university-of-pennsylvania-classification-of-osteonecrosis/.
69. Yawn BP, Buchanan GR, Afenyi-Annan AN, et al. Management of sickle cell disease: summary of the 2014 evidence-based report by expert panel members. JAMA 2014;312(10):1033–48.
70. Marti-Carvajal AJ, Sola I, Agreda-Perez LH. Treatment for avascular necrosis of bone in people with sickle cell disease. Cochrane Database Syst Rev 2019; 12(12):CD004344.
71. Osunkwo I. An update on the recent literature on sickle cell bone disease. Curr Opin Endocrinol Diabetes Obes 2013;20(6):539–46.
72. Chen CH, Chang JK, Lai KA, et al. Alendronate in the prevention of collapse of the femoral head in nontraumatic osteonecrosis: a two-year multicenter, prospective, randomized, double-blind, placebo-controlled study. Arthritis Rheum 2012; 64(5):1572–8.
73. Lai KA, Shen WJ, Yang CY, et al. The use of alendronate to prevent early collapse of the femoral head in patients with nontraumatic osteonecrosis. A randomized clinical study. J Bone Joint Surg 2005;87(10):2155–9.
74. Lee YK, Ha YC, Cho YJ, et al. Does Zoledronate Prevent Femoral Head Collapse from Osteonecrosis? A Prospective, Randomized, Open-Label, Multicenter Study. J Bone Joint Surg 2015;97(14):1142–8.

75. Arai R, Takahashi D, Inoue M, et al. Efficacy of teriparatide in the treatment of non-traumatic osteonecrosis of the femoral head: a retrospective comparative study with alendronate. BMC Musculoskelet Disord 2017;18(1):24.
76. Grimbly C, Escagedo PD, Jaremko JL, et al. Sickle cell bone disease and response to intravenous bisphosphonates in children. Osteoporos Int 2022; 33(11):2397–408.
77. Marom R, Rabenhorst BM, Morello R. Osteogenesis imperfecta: an update on clinical features and therapies. Eur J Endocrinol 2020;183(4):R95–106.
78. Miller RG, Segal JB, Ashar BH, et al. High prevalence and correlates of low bone mineral density in young adults with sickle cell disease. Am J Hematol 2006; 81(4):236–41.
79. Wright NC, Looker AC, Saag KG, et al. The recent prevalence of osteoporosis and low bone mass in the United States based on bone mineral density at the femoral neck or lumbar spine. J Bone Miner Res 2014;29(11):2520–6.
80. Giordano P, Urbano F, Lassandro G, et al. Mechanisms of Bone Impairment in Sickle Bone Disease. Int J Environ Res Public Health 2021;(4):18. https://doi.org/10.3390/ijerph18041832.
81. Ross AC, Manson JE, Abrams SA, et al. The 2011 report on dietary reference intakes for calcium and vitamin D from the Institute of Medicine: what clinicians need to know. J Clin Endocrinol Metab 2011;96(1):53–8.
82. Herrick KA, Storandt RJ, Afful J, et al. Vitamin D status in the United States, 2011-2014. Am J Clin Nutr 2019;110(1):150–7.
83. Forrest KY, Stuhldreher WL. Prevalence and correlates of vitamin D deficiency in US adults. Nutr Res 2011;31(1):48–54.
84. Nolan VG, Nottage KA, Cole EW, et al. Prevalence of vitamin D deficiency in sickle cell disease: a systematic review. PLoS One 2015;10(3):e0119908.
85. Buison AM, Kawchak DA, Schall J, et al. Low vitamin D status in children with sickle cell disease. J Pediatr 2004;145(5):622–7.
86. Rovner AJ, Stallings VA, Kawchak DA, et al. High risk of vitamin D deficiency in children with sickle cell disease. J Am Diet Assoc 2008;108(9):1512–6.
87. Burnett-Bowie SM, Cappola AR. The USPSTF 2021 Recommendations on Screening for Asymptomatic Vitamin D Deficiency in Adults: The Challenge for Clinicians Continues. JAMA 2021;325(14):1401–2.
88. Soe HH, Abas AB, Than NN, et al. Vitamin D supplementation for sickle cell disease. Cochrane Database Syst Rev 2017;1(1):CD010858.
89. Arlet JB, Courbebaisse M, Chatellier G, et al. Relationship between vitamin D deficiency and bone fragility in sickle cell disease: a cohort study of 56 adults. Bone 2013;52(1):206–11.
90. De Franceschi L, Gabbiani D, Giusti A, et al. Development of algorithm for clinical management of sickle cell bone disease: evidence for a role of vertebral fractures in patient follow-up. J Clin Med 2020;9(5). https://doi.org/10.3390/jcm9051601.

Global Health Disparities in Childhood Rickets

Alicia Diaz-Thomas, MD, MPH[a,*], Pallavi Iyer, MD[b]

KEYWORDS

- Health disparities • Rickets • Vitamin D deficiency

KEY POINTS

- Addressing health disparities in care of global rickets is important in delaying and preventing adult osteoporosis.
- Nutritional rickets is a due to calcium or vitamin D deficiency caused by sub-optimal nutrition and/or ultraviolet light exposure.
- Biological, sociocultural, and geo-environmental barriers impact the recognition, prevention, and treatment of rickets in vulnerable populations.
- Global policies and investments are needed to eradicate rickets.

INTRODUCTION

Osteoporosis is a disease with its origins in childhood. Bone mass attained early in life is perhaps the most important determinant in lifelong skeletal health; growth in bone size and strength occurs in childhood and is complete by the third decade of life. Thus, the accrual of peak bone mass is largely a pediatric and young adult phenomenon. A 10% increase in peak bone mass gain can have significant influence on risk reduction of osteoporosis later in life; and in one analysis, postponed onset of osteoporosis by 13 years.[1,2] Suboptimal peak bone mass may be related to not only osteoporosis in later life but also fractures in childhood and adolescence.[3]

Acquisition of peak bone mass is a function of not only genetics, but also sex and environment and is thus subject to health disparities as a function of race/ethnicity. Prematurity, poor nutrition regardless of body mass index, food insecurity, decreased

Disclaimers: It is important to note that we use the terms women and breastfeeding for brevity; we recognize that not all people who breastfeed or chest feed identify as women.

[a] Department of Pediatrics, Division of Pediatric Endocrinology, The University of Tennessee Health Science Center, 910 Madison Avenue, Suite 1010, Memphis, TN 38163, USA; [b] Department of Pediatrics, Division of Endocrinology and Diabetes, Medical College of Wisconsin, Children's Corporate Center, Suite 520, 9000 West Wisconsin Avenue, Milwaukee, WI 53226, USA

* Corresponding author. UTHSC-Memphis, Room 1006, 910 Madison Avenue, Memphis, TN 38163.

E-mail address: adiaztho@uthsc.edu

Endocrinol Metab Clin N Am 52 (2023) 643–657
https://doi.org/10.1016/j.ecl.2023.05.011

access to opportunities for physical activity, decreased access to sufficient sunlight, and lack of awareness by health care providers and governments who control health programs serve to worsen health outcomes in a race/ethnicity/socioeconomic class-based fashion.

Osteoporosis and osteoporotic fractures are set to increase in the coming decades as globally, our population ages. Osteomalacia, decreased mineralization of bone in a mature skeleton resulting in increased osteoid, is also widespread and radiographically on dual-energy X-ray absorptiometry, can present with low bone mineral density. Osteomalacia and osteoporosis can be confounded or can coexist, but both cause significant disability and pain.[4] Climate change has also caused significant environmental and subsequent agricultural and economic challenges. The role of environmental factors in osteoporosis, such as air pollution, is being investigated.[5,6] Exposure to famine at early stages in life (gestation to adolescence) is associated with increased risk of osteoporosis or osteoporotic fracture.[7]

Nutritional rickets is a condition of a growing child due to calcium or vitamin D deficiency—either from nutritional sources or through ultraviolet B (UVB) rays induced endogenous vitamin D production. Rickets may be an early marker for increased risks of osteomalacia or osteoporosis later in life due to the decreased mineralization of bone itself. In this article, we will discuss how the interplay between nutrition, environment, economics, and race/ethnicity results in health disparities in pediatric nutritional rickets.

RICKETS

Rickets is a condition characterized by impaired bone mineralization at the growth plates in infants and children. Physiologically, it represents a disorder of defective chondrocyte differentiation, decreased mineralization of the growth plate, and defective osteoid mineralization. Physical findings include skeletal deformity, growth stunting, muscular weakness, and if untreated, can lead to lifelong skeletal deformity, osteomalacia, developmental delays, and impaired motor function. These can have serious consequences in adulthood for a person's lifelong professional and personal well-being leading to chronic pain and disability both of which may be limiting for a person's function in the workplace.

Rickets is usually caused by a lack of either of the 2 important mineral components of bone, phosphorus (phosphopenic) or calcium (calcipenic); most rickets is the calcipenic form. Although rickets can have many causes, some of which are genetic, most rickets is what is described as nutritional, either from deficiency of 25(OH)D (25-hydroxy vitamin D) and/or from calcium insufficiency. Nutritional rickets is present globally and social determinants of health including social, economic, political, and religious factors lead to health disparities in care of calcium and vitamin D deficient rickets.

Rickets is one of the most common global childhood conditions. In the United Kingdom (UK), where rickets has a long history in medical care, low concentrations of serum 25(OH)D are common during the winter months in all ethnic groups[8] with higher frequency reported in Southeast Asian, African, and Afro-Caribbean immigrant communities. Similarly, low vitamin D status and rickets are more prevalent in immigrant children in the Netherlands, Denmark, Norway, Spain, Australia, and New Zealand.[9–15] Reports of biochemical osteomalacia and rickets in the Middle East also note a relatively high prevalence: 10% of Arab adolescents in Saudi Arabia, 27% of Yemeni infants in another, and 23% of Turkish children in a particular region of Turkey have been described.[12–14] In India, the use of purdah (facial to full-body covering) among

Muslims results in rickets rates 3 to 4 times higher than among Hindu girls.[16] Among children and infants in China, prevalence rate of rickets is 15.9% (<5 years old), and 26.7% (infants) with rural north-east China reporting rates of clinical rickets in 0 to 2 years old as 49.3%.[17] Reports of rickets are also found in Bangladesh, Pakistan, North Korea, and Japan. Nutritional rickets in Africa occurs predominantly in settings of low dietary calcium intakes and has been described in both northern and southern areas. In North America, rickets has been described most frequently in breastfed infants and in children receiving calcium restricted/deficient diets. In Argentina, southernmost areas farthest away from the equator report vitamin D deficiency rickets whereas areas of Uruguay attribute etiology to calcium deficiency in diet.[18]

Epidemiological data show that hypocalcemia and rickets due to vitamin D deficiency are not usually diagnosed until weeks to months after birth; the peak incidence is between 6 and 18 months, even in regions where vitamin D deficiency is endemic.[19–22] After the age of 2 years, calcium deficiency rickets is more common and often associated with weaning from breastfeeding.[17] Maternal calcium and vitamin D deficiency predispose infants to increased risks of hypocalcemia and development of rickets over time. Exclusively breastfed infants, who do not themselves receive vitamin D supplementation, may also develop rickets. Once weaned, infants not receiving sufficient dietary calcium may develop hypocalcemia, secondary hyperparathyroidism, and rickets.

These vulnerable populations—pregnant women, infants, and children—have risks that are dictated by factors out of their control and serve to illustrate how their experiences in the social and nutritional determinants of health lead to the health disparities in the incidence and prevalence of rickets. Geopolitical factors such as migration from equatorial regions to higher latitudes, practices that increase body coverage with

	Nutrition	Sun exposure
Biological	Lactose intolerance Prematurity Maternal health effects on fetus	Melanin density on the skin
Socio-cultural	Diets rich in phytic acid Special diets poor in calcium, vitamin D Lack of access to nutritious food	Clothing coverage Use of SPF lotions Pollution Crowded housing, tall buildings
Geo-environmental	Famine Climate Change	Human trafficking and migration to higher latitudes

Fig. 1. Schematic of biological, sociocultural, and geo-environmental barriers that affect nutritional stores of calcium and vitamin D and cutaneous production of vitamin D.

clothes/sun protection factor (SPF) emollients, decreased access to open/pollution-free environments, or poor nutrition have led to these disparities (**Fig. 1**).

Historical Context of Rickets

Historically, rickets has been often described in more marginalized populations with limited sun exposure (movement to urban indoor spaces, living in high smog areas, migration/forced movement of dark-pigmented individuals from equatorial UV light exposure to higher latitudes, wearing clothing that covers most of the body) or due to poor nutrition (lack of access to adequate vitamin-D rich diets or fortified foods). Although the description of rachitic changes in children has been described for centuries, the first systematic publication of rickets was in 1645, and further characterized in 1650 after studying English children that were primarily indoors and working as wool spinners. Increased incidence of rickets was observed during the northern European industrial revolution from the 17th to the 20th century where poor children were concentrated in urban areas with increased smog and perhaps decreased sources of dairy.[23] In the 1800s, it was suggested that sunlight may be preventive in developing rickets as it was noted that children from tropical countries were less likely to have rickets than those in northern Europe. In 1916, Alfred Hess and LI Unger undertook a study in New York to study the effects of cod liver oil in preventing rickets. They noted that "of all races, the negro is most subject to rickets." This study led to establishing a center for maternal and childcare in New York to combat rickets.[24,25] Similarly in England at the same time, Edward Mellanby showed that along with sunlight, nutritional supplementation with cod liver oil, milk, or butter could prevent rickets. Soon it was verified that vitamin D could be either synthesized in the skin or ingested. During World War II, the British government ran state-run cafeterias to increase access to nutritious food and fortifying margarine with vitamin D along with providing special diets for expectant mothers and toddlers,[26] leading to a drastic decrease in incidence of nutritional rickets.

However, there was an uptick of the disease in the 1960s to 1970s in England and was noted mostly in recent immigrants from Commonwealth countries from South Asia. Presence of high concentration of melanin is noted in people closer to the equator where there is high UV radiation from the sun, as melanin is protective against UV radiation damage, but allows for conversion of 7-dehydrocholesterol to active vitamin D.[27] The reemergence of rickets in England in the 1970s was labeled as Asian rickets, and these migrants were blamed for the disease rather than recognizing that it was a consequence of poor environment in urban areas.[26]

Migration of people with melanin-rich skin from equatorial latitudes to higher latitudes can also lead to higher incidence of rickets. These patterns have been seen with the forced trafficking of humans from Africa to America during slave trades, refugees escaping war-torn countries, or emigration of families due to economic constraints or to seek better opportunities. In an Australian study using X-ray evidence of rickets, higher rates were found in those migrating from the Indian subcontinent (37%), Africa (33%), and the Middle East (11%).[10] In the UK, incidence and prevalence of rickets has been increasing, particularly among African and South Asian migrant populations.[28] In a population-based study performed over 40 years in Olmsted County, Minnesota, USA, the incidence of nutritional rickets in children younger than 3 years increased over 200% from 1970 to 2000, with the highest increases coinciding with the emigration of Somali refugees to the county.[29] In a review of case reports of rickets from 1986 to 2003 in the United States, the vast majority of cases were in breastfed non-Hispanic black (NHB) children who had not received vitamin D supplementation.[30]

Pregnancy and Fetal Life

Fetal bone and mineral metabolism are regulated differently from postnatal life. In fetal life, the placenta actively "pumps" calcium, phosphorus, and magnesium against electrochemical and concentration gradients in a parathyroid hormone (PTH) and parathyroid hormone related peptide (PTHrP)-mediated fashion.[21] This allows for the rapid mineralization of bone, the majority of which occurs in the third trimester. This is considered a vitamin D independent process, and thus maternal vitamin D deficiency, unless severe, is not expected to cause rickets in fetal life.[21] This physiologic mechanism also protects the fetus against maternal calcium deficiency in all but the most extreme cases.

Recent evidence suggests that vitamin D deficiency is common during pregnancy especially among high-risk groups, including vegetarians, women with limited sun exposure (eg, those who live in cold climates, reside in northern latitudes, or wear sun and winter protective clothing), and ethnic minorities (South Asian, African/African descendants, and Middle Eastern), especially those with darker skin (https://www.acog.org/clinical/clinical-guidance/committee-opinion/articles/2011/07/vitamin-d-screening-and-supplementation-during-pregnancy). The 2016 Global Consensus Recommendations on Prevention and Management of Nutritional Rickets recommends that women of childbearing age protect themselves against vitamin D deficiency.[31] In regions where sunlight is limited and diet does not include foods high in vitamin D, maternal deficiency leads to extremely low vitamin D in newborns and breastfed children.[32]

There is no current recommendation for vitamin D screening in pregnancy, although screening for risk factors may prompt biochemical screening or therapeutic intervention of pregnant women. In 2010, the Food and Nutrition Board at the Institute of Medicine of the National Academies established that an adequate intake of vitamin D during pregnancy and lactation was 600 international units per day. Most prenatal vitamins typically contain 400 international units of vitamin D per tablet. However, the threshold of optimal serum level of vitamin D sufficiency remains an area of active research in pregnant women.

Although there is no evidence that maternal vitamin supplementation improves birth size of a newborn, neonatal vitamin D stores reflect maternal vitamin D levels found in cord blood and may play a role in improving intestinal calcium absorption in early infant life and avoiding complications of neonatal hypocalcemia which can be life threatening.[28,33] In one example, Brooke and colleagues[34] performed a double-blind placebo-controlled trial involving late third trimester supplementation of Asian women with severe vitamin D deficiency with 1000 IU daily of 25(OH)D, and noted no statistically significant change in anthropomorphic measurements, but 5 infants in the control group had symptomatic hypocalcemia without radiographic evidence of rickets.

Neonatal and Infant Life

In the immediate postnatal period, there is a switch in the regulation of mineral homeostasis that occurs as calcium levels fall postnatally (due to loss of the placenta). This is followed by a rise in parathyroid hormone followed by an increase in 1,25-dihydroxyvitamin D: $1,25(OH)_2D$. Phosphorus metabolism also changes, regulated by fibroblast growth factor-23 (FGF23). Initially, intestinal absorption of calcium is mostly passive and facilitated by lactose.[21] Over the next few weeks to months, intestinal calcium absorption increasingly transitions from a passive to an active process, requiring the actions of $1,25\text{-}(OH)_2D$, and thus dependent on 25(OH)D concentrations. Rickets may develop in infancy if vitamin D and mineral deficiencies continue.

Preterm infants

Preterm infants are at an even more risk of having vitamin D deficiency/rickets due to lower 25(OH)D stores resulting from shorter time of placental vitamin D transfer, reduced calcium stores, stress of concomitant illness, reduced mobility and sun-exposure in the neonatal intensive care unit, and need for parenteral feeds. The incidence of metabolic bone disease occurs in 30% to 50% of preterm infants.[35] The incidence of delivering a preterm (32–37 weeks) and very preterm (<32 weeks) infant is higher in black versus white mothers. The variables that contribute most to these disparities are maternal level of education, marital status/paternity knowledge, type of medical insurance, and maternal hypertension.[36] Not only is there a higher proportion of preterm births in NHB compared to non-Hispanic whites (NHW), but there is also an increased incidence of recurrent preterm birth in this population.[37] This leads to a disproportionate burden of rickets in premature infants of mothers of NHB compared with NHW.

Feeding practices

Breastfeeding is the preferred form of infant nutrition, providing health benefits for the infant–mother pair in addition to being cost-effective,[38] but provides a lower concentration of vitamin D then commercial formulas. The World Health Organization (WHO) recommends exclusive breastfeeding for the first 6 months of life, and continued breastfeeding for at least the first 2 years of life, with complementary foods being introduced at 6 months post-partum (WHO. Breastfeeding 2021. https://www.who.int/health-topics/breastfeeding#tab=tab_1) (accessed Feb 26, 2023). However, structural barriers to breastfeeding include gender inequities, pressure from commercial entities to promote other infant feeding practices, breastfeeding averse sociocultural infant feeding norms, labor markets and health care systems whose practices do not promote breastfeeding, and economic policies that constrain public health systems.[39,40] Even when breast milk is the primary source of infant nutrition, the concomitant vitamin D supplementation for the infant is not always emphasized. Barriers to breastfeeding can mirror to those related to infant nutrition and prevention of conditions such as rickets.

Even infants who primarily drink infant formula are at risk for vitamin D deficiency. Currently, infant formulas in United States are only required to have a minimum of 400 IU vitamin D per liter. Generally, infants younger than 6 months drink about 500 mL of formula per day and thus receive only 200 IU vitamin D/day. Therefore, the American Academy of Pediatrics (AAP) recommends that infants consuming less than 500 mL of formula daily be supplemented with vitamin D.[41]

It is especially important to recognize that families that avoid medical care, vaccines, or certain medications may be at a higher risk of not receiving adequate counseling on vitamin D supplementation which is especially important in primarily breastfed infants who when supplemented with table food follow a vegan diet.[42,43]

Sun exposure

Amount of sunlight required to prevent vitamin D deficiency in infants varies by the latitude, season, time of day, air quality, amount of skin melanin density, and amount of skin exposed to sunlight. Thus, an infant's environment directly contributes to vitamin D sufficiency and may reflect the inequities perpetuated by the built environment. For comparison of similar latitudes around 40°, one study in Cincinnati showed that 20 min/d of exposure to hands and face generated enough sun exposure to increase vitamin D concentration, but in Beijing, 2 h/d of exposure was needed to increase vitamin D concentration likely due to increased pollution in China. For exclusively breastfed infants younger than 6 months, 30 minutes per week of sun exposure is needed if wearing only a diaper.[44] These studies do not comment on the melanin coverage in these babies. However to reduce the risk of skin cancer, the AAP recommends avoiding direct sunlight in infants younger than 6 months.[45] Thus along with nutritional components, disparities in UVB ray exposure can place infants at a higher risk of vitamin D deficiency and rickets.

Vitamin D supplementation

The vitamin D content of breastmilk is low, comprising approximately 3 IU/100 g (https://fdc.nal.usda.gov/fdc-app.html#/food-details/171279/nutrients) (accessed on Feb 26, 2023). The relationship between early life feedings and later adult bone health is unclear and understudied and may be confounded by rates of vitamin D sufficiency.[22,46,47] As breastfeeding rates rise to levels proposed by the WHO, supplementation of breastfed infants will become increasingly important. Thus, implementation of breastfeeding promotion and attention to promotion of appropriate supplementation should occur in tandem.

Infants and toddlers are at highest risk for serious complications from vitamin D deficiency and hypocalcemia. They may present with hypocalcemic seizures, dilated cardiomyopathy, dysrhythmia, and rickets.[48] In a 2-year prospective British study using the British Pediatric Surveillance Unit, the incidence of hypocalcemic seizure was 3.9 per 1 million children aged 0 to 15 years with infant males of South Asian or black heritage noted to have the highest incidence rates. Notably, 19% of the cases were found in formula fed infants, pointing to the need for universal supplementation. In a Turkish study of late neonatal hypocalcemia, the prevalence of vitamin D deficiency (defined as <12 ng/mL) was high in both the neonates (86.5%) and mothers (93%).[49] Iranian and Korean studies found a positive correlation between late neonatal hypocalcemia and maternal vitamin D deficiency.[50,51]

Importantly, for rickets prevention, programs that encourage and promote breastfeeding need to include education about vitamin D supplementation. Nutritional rickets in exclusively breastfed children is not rare in the United States, with reports citing that up to 70% of children with nutritional rickets are exclusively breastfed without vitamin D supplementation.[30] In an analysis of the 2009 to 2016 National Health and Nutrition Examination Survey (NHANES) dataset, less than 40% of US infants received appropriate vitamin D supplementation in nearly all demographic subgroups, despite the AAP 2008 guidelines on Vitamin D intake recommending supplementation.[52] Despite having national policies for infant vitamin D supplementation in Europe, adherence varies with the UK having the lowest rates of vitamin D supplementation.[53]

Childhood

Failure to attain one's genetically programmed bone mass occurs when calcium intake is insufficient during growth. Despite the importance of childhood and adolescent calcium intake in preventing adult-onset osteoporosis, there are few studies evaluating calcium intake and skeletal status in children when compared to adult studies. In one meta-analysis of 139 studies published in English, only 22% of the studies were pediatric in nature.[54] Low calcium intake is often reported in adolescents, older adults, and in those people with a low income residing in a high-income country (HIC) as well as residents of Asia, Africa, and Latin America.[55] Meta-analysis of studies reporting calcium intake of pregnant women included 73,958 women in 37 countries, calcium intake during pregnancy was less than 800 mg/d in 29% of the HIC's and 82% of the low and middle income countries (LMICs) represented.[56] Reviewing NHANES

2009 to 2012 datasets revealed that levels of calcium along with other nutrients were lowest among NHB when compared to NHW and Hispanics even when accounting for the poverty index ratio. Despite the importance of childhood and adolescent calcium intake in preventing adult-onset osteoporosis, there are few studies evaluating calcium intake and skeletal status in children when compared to adult studies. Optimal intake is achieved through diet, supplementation, or a combination of the two.[57]

Decreased availability of calcium rich foods

In 1978, John Pettifor and colleagues[58] described a group of South African children with nutritional rickets who had normal vitamin D levels. These children were placed on a calcium rich diet and rickets resolved. The description of calcipenic rickets in vitamin D sufficient individuals has been since described in equatorial regions and in children with restricted diets.[59,60] Inadequate dietary calcium is a global health problem, disproportionately affecting LMICs. Its roots lie in a myriad of spaces including availability of calcium rich foods, bioavailability of the calcium within those foods, availability and accessibility of calcium supplementation, and population characteristics that include vitamin D status.[61] Assessment of population level calcium sufficiency can be challenging, and thus epidemiological data are lacking.[61]

Calcium is found in high quantities in dairy foods, but much of the world's countries do not rely on dairy as a source of calcium. In developed countries, dairy foods account for approximately 14% of the total dietary energy intake, but in LMICs, these foods represent a mere 4% of dietary energy intake.[62] Furthermore, widespread lactose intolerance makes this an inappropriate source of calcium for many populations.[62] Overall in countries with historically low dairy intake such as China and India, there has been a steady increase in consumption of dairy products, but it has not correlated with an increase in calcium intake, and there are growing concerns of environmental effects of increased dairy production globally.[63]

Prevalence of phytates in diet

Calcium intakes of 200 to 300 mg/d have been reported from Egypt, Kenya, Nigeria, Gambia, and South Africa. In these areas, not only is there a minimal intake of dairy products, but the diets are rich in substances that reduce the bioavailability of calcium. Phytic acid (a calcium-binder) found in grains, oxalates in green leaves, tannic acid in tea, and saturated fat in palm oil inhibit absorption of ingested calcium and are commonly consumed in Africa.[64–67] Unleavened breads like chappatti and raghif eaten in South Asia and Middle East are also rich in phytic acid interfering with calcium absorption. Soy-based formulas often used in infancy also contain phytic acid and have a lower calcium/phosphate ratio.[35]

Another confounding public health factor is fluorosis. A study of 400,000 children in rural India reported that 45% of the drinking water sources had a high fluoride content (1.5–25 ppm). Excess fluoride exacerbates calcium deficiency, leading to skeletal fluorosis with rachitic symptoms. This disorder was more prevalent among children with low calcium intakes but present even when serum calcium and vitamin D levels were in the normal range.[68,69]

Lack of exposure to ultraviolet radiation

As noted earlier, vitamin D is also manufactured by human skin exposed to ultraviolet radiation, and changes in UVB exposure related to multiple reasons can lead to vitamin D deficiency and increased risks of rickets. The amount of UV rays to which one is exposed occurs as a function of the angle at which solar radiation passes through the atmosphere, the mass of air through which the sun's rays must pass, and the presence of clouds and pollution in the lower atmosphere.[70] Time of day, season, latitude, clothing, and other behaviors further complicate the equation. People living in urban environments may experience not only air pollution, but also the effects of tall buildings blocking out sunlight. Because of risk of skin cancer, use of SPF lotions and SPF blocking clothing has increased. Using sunscreens with SPF of as little as 8 SPF dramatically reduces endogenous vitamin D production by 95%.[71] There are also people due to personal preference or due to socioreligious norms who choose to wear clothes that fully cover their bodies limiting sun exposure and thus cutaneous vitamin D production.

Solutions

There are no screening guidelines to measure vitamin D values, but rather to screen populations for risk of calcium and vitamin D deficiency and prescribe/recommend calcium and vitamin D supplementation accordingly. Refugee infants and children (less than 6 years of age) should be provided with a multivitamin that includes recommended daily allowances for vitamin D. Refugee children older than 6 years of age with clinical or laboratory evidence of poor nutrition should also receive supplementation (https://www.cdc.gov/immigrantrefugeehealth/guidelines/domestic/nutrition-growth.html).

Universal supplementation of vitamin D

Probable impediments to meeting the AAP guidelines for vitamin D supplementation in infants include a combination of inconsistent prescribing by clinicians and poor adherence to the use of a supplement by parents of infants, and it is further complicated by a lack of awareness of the consequences of vitamin D deficiency in infants among the public.[72]

Even when vitamin D supplementation is appropriately prescribed, government or commercial funded insurance programs may not cover these supplements. In the United States, the Women Infant Children nutrition program is a food program but is unable to distribute any supplements. Vitamin D is an approved Medicaid supplement but requires a health care provider prescription,[73] further limiting implementation of this therapeutic intervention. Thoughtful discussions should be undertaken to address family preferences regarding the source of vitamin D as several formulations are available: plant based, fish-oil based, animal-based gelatins, and Halal certified pork-free vitamin D supplements. Other concerns include palatability of vitamin D supplements and lack of insurance coverage in the United States for calcium supplementation (author experience).

In a survey conducted by the European Society of Pediatric Endocrinology Bone and Growth Plate working group, nearly 97% of all European countries reported having a national policy for infant vitamin D supplementation. Some factors associated with good adherence to this policy include universal supplementation independent of feeding mode, education on supplementation prior to discharge from the nursery, providing financial support for purchase of supplements, and monitoring adherence at follow-up visits. Countries that included one or more of the protective factors had higher rates of sustained supplementation.[53]

- It is important to remember that there are several formulations of vitamin D supplements and different families may prefer one over another. Investigators in Canada found that parents preferred either 400 IU of vitamin D provided in dissolving filmstrips or concentrated vitamin D administered as 1 drop to 1 mL of liquid administered by a dropper.[74,75] Data suggest that supplementing mothers of exclusively breastfed infants with vitamin D can provide adequate levels of vitamin D in infants in the first month of life, but more research is needed.[76]

- In LMICs with a higher prevalence of vitamin D deficiency than the United States, a public health approach has included mandatory fortification of staple foods in addition to supplementation of at-risk subgroups.[77]

Fortification with calcium

Food fortification has been identified as the most cost-effective strategy to overcome micronutrient deficiencies. Currently, 130 countries have mandatory supplementation of salt with iodine, and 85 countries fortify wheat flour with micronutrients such as iron, iodine, folate, and vitamin A.[78] Fortified foods should be widely available and readily accepted by the at-risk population to be successful in irradicating deficiencies.[55]

Agricultural subsidies are an important factor for influencing food production; they should be able to positively influence a system that in many high and middle income country (HMICs) is currently neither healthful nor sustainable.[79] Replacing animal sourced foods with plant-based foods can have significant effects toward global reduction of environmental impacts and improve health of many populations.[80] However, attention needs to be paid to adequacy of vitamin D and calcium in such diets.

Calcium fortification of foods can be limited by the low bioavailability of calcium salts, the decreased solubility in certain food products, the possibility of changing the taste or appearance of the food, and the differing amounts needed in different population groups. Nevertheless, given the lack of adequate calcium-rich diets, particularly in LMICs, fortification of foods with calcium should be considered. Examples of nontraditional experimental sources of calcium for food fortification include powders made from eggshells or bones of tuna and calcium derived from algae.[81] Caution must be taken to coordinate efforts with a country or region such that the fortification of many different food sources does not cause overconsumption and is mindful of regional dietary preferences. The WHO has software programs that can assist with estimation of amount of fortification required to target desired degree of supplementation. Mandatory or mass fortification of foods usually requires a centralized production or legislation of smaller manufacturers.[55] The WHO and the Food and Agriculture Organization (FAO) have a framework for evaluating and monitoring calcium fortified foods (WHO FAO Guidelines on food fortification 2006; https://www.who.int/publications/i/item/9241594012). There are also tools available for the assessment of data on quality coverage and consumption of fortified foods across countries (www.gainhealth.org).

Fortification with vitamin D

In the European Union, the beneficial effects of this strategy are limited due to a restriction of the maximum content of vitamin D in livestock feed (https://eur-lex.europa.eu/legal-content/EN/TXT/?uri=CELEX%3A52004XC0225%2803%29. Accessed Feb 26, 2023). However, apart from this limitation, it is still possible to increase the content of vitamin D in food of animal origin. Examples exist in terms of increasing the vitamin D content of feed for pigs and hens. In the latter case, egg content of vitamin D could be markedly increased.

More rigorous trials

Despite our knowledge of nutritional rickets and its determinants, a recent Cochrane review examining the effects of vitamin D, calcium, or a combination of vitamin D and calcium for the treatment of nutritional rickets in children found only 4 randomized controlled trial (RCTs) out of 4562 studies with 2 studies conducted in Nigeria and 2 in India. The authors concluded that based on the paucity of data, they were unable to make specific recommendations to best treatment regimens for treatment of nutritional rickets.[82] For a condition with such a wide-ranging burden of disease, adequately designed randomized controlled trials are critical in establishing the optimal dose and duration of vitamin D and calcium supplementation in preventing/treating multiple health outcomes (rickets healing, peak bone mass, risk of fracture) in global populations. In addition, a worldwide initiative is needed to eradicate rickets, acknowledging the disproportionate burden of this disease globally in marginalized people, which could be spearheaded by the WHO in much the same fashion as has been done for iodine deficiency.[83]

SUMMARY

Recognition and treatment of nutritional rickets and osteomalacia in infancy and childhood can help prevent or delay adult osteoporosis. Health disparities rooted in race, gender, socioeconomic status, and geopolitical factors result in disproportionate burden of a preventable disease such as rickets in vulnerable populations. Acknowledging these differences can help inform best policies and invest in global solutions to prevent childhood rickets and eliminate disparities in bone health.

CLINICS CARE POINTS

- Prevention of morbidity associated with osteoporosis with global health policies and financial resources to prevent nutritional rickets starts in childhood.
- In marginalized populations of pregnant women, infants, and children – recent refugees and people who have migrated from equatorial to higher latitudes – are at an increased risk for nutritional rickets due to generational-systematic factors. A careful assessment of social determinants of health is helpful in considering need for supplementation with vitamin D.
- Globally, education and resources to assure adequate vitamin D supplementation in breastfed and premature infants is vital in preventing nutritional rickets.

DISCLOSURE

The authors have no commercial or financial conflicts of interest. No grant funds were provided for the preparation of the article.

REFERENCES

1. Hernandez CJ, Beaupre GS, Carter DR. A theoretical analysis of the relative influences of peak BMD, age-related bone loss and menopause on the development of osteoporosis. Osteoporos Int 2003;14(10):843–7.
2. Zhu X, Zheng H. Factors influencing peak bone mass gain. Front Med 2021;15(1):53–69.
3. Nih Consensus Development Panel on Osteoporosis Prevention D, Therapy. Osteoporosis prevention, diagnosis, and therapy. JAMA 2001;285(6):785–95.
4. Cianferotti L. Osteomalacia Is Not a Single Disease. Int J Mol Sci 2022;23(23). https://doi.org/10.3390/ijms232314896.
5. Mousavibaygei SR, Bisadi A, ZareSakhvidi F. Outdoor air pollution exposure, bone mineral density, osteoporosis, and osteoporotic fractures: A systematic review and meta-analysis. Sci Total Environ 2023;865:161117.
6. Prada D, Crandall CJ, Kupsco A, et al. Air pollution and decreased bone mineral density among Women's Health Initiative participants. EClinicalMedicine 2023;57:101864.

7. Yang M, Yin H, Zhen D, et al. Exposure to famine in every stage of life and the risk of osteoporosis and fractures later in life: A cross-sectional study. Bone 2023;168: 116644.
8. Lawson M, Thomas M. Vitamin D concentrations in Asian children aged 2 years living in England: population survey. BMJ 1999;318(7175):28.
9. Pedersen P, Michaelsen KF, Molgaard C. Children with nutritional rickets referred to hospitals in Copenhagen during a 10-year period. Acta Paediatr 2003;92(1): 87–90.
10. Robinson PD, Hogler W, Craig ME, et al. The re-emerging burden of rickets: a decade of experience from Sydney. Arch Dis Child 2006;91(7):564–8.
11. Yeste D, Carrascosa A. [Nutritional rickets in childhood: analysis of 62 cases]. Med Clin 2003;121(1):23–7. Raquitismo carencial en la infancia: analisis de 62 casos.
12. Narchi H, El Jamil M, Kulaylat N. Symptomatic rickets in adolescence. Arch Dis Child 2001;84(6):501–3.
13. Ozgur S, Sumer H, Kocoglu G. Rickets and soil strontium. Arch Dis Child 1996; 75(6):524–6.
14. Underwood P, Margetts B. High levels of childhood rickets in rural North Yemen. Soc Sci Med 1987;24(1):37–41.
15. Al-Daghri NM, Yakout S, Sabico S, et al. Establishing the Prevalence of Osteomalacia in Arab Adolescents Using Biochemical Markers of Bone Health. Nutrients 2022;14(24). https://doi.org/10.3390/nu14245354.
16. Bhattacharyya AK. Nutritional rickets in the tropics. World Rev Nutr Diet 1992;67: 140–97.
17. Thacher TD, Fischer PR, Strand MA, et al. Nutritional rickets around the world: causes and future directions. Ann Trop Paediatr 2006;26(1):1–16.
18. Oliveri MB, Ladizesky M, Mautalen CA, et al. Seasonal variations of 25 hydroxyvitamin D and parathyroid hormone in Ushuaia (Argentina), the southernmost city of the world. Bone Miner 1993;20(1):99–108.
19. Al-Mustafa ZH, Al-Madan M, Al-Majid HJ, et al. Vitamin D deficiency and rickets in the Eastern Province of Saudi Arabia. Ann Trop Paediatr 2007;27(1):63–7.
20. Beck-Nielsen SS, Brock-Jacobsen B, Gram J, et al. Incidence and prevalence of nutritional and hereditary rickets in southern Denmark. Eur J Endocrinol 2009; 160(3):491–7.
21. Kovacs CS. Bone development and mineral homeostasis in the fetus and neonate: roles of the calciotropic and phosphotropic hormones. Physiol Rev 2014;94(4):1143–218.
22. Pereira GR, Zucker AH. Nutritional deficiencies in the neonate. Clin Perinatol 1986;13(1):175–89.
23. Shore RM, Chesney RW. Rickets: Part I. Pediatr Radiol 2013;43(2):140–51.
24. Rajakumar K, Thomas SB. Reemerging nutritional rickets: a historical perspective. Arch Pediatr Adolesc Med 2005;159(4):335–41.
25. Wheeler BJ, Snoddy AME, Munns C, et al. A Brief History of Nutritional Rickets. Front Endocrinol 2019;10:795.
26. Bivins R. Ideology and disease identity: the politics of rickets, 1929-1982. Med Humanit 2014;40(1):3–10.
27. Ames BN, Grant WB, Willett WC. Does the High Prevalence of Vitamin D Deficiency in African Americans Contribute to Health Disparities? Nutrients 2021; 13(2). https://doi.org/10.3390/nu13020499.
28. Uday S, Hogler W. Prevention of rickets and osteomalacia in the UK: political action overdue. Arch Dis Child 2018;103(9):901–6.

29. Thacher TD, Fischer PR, Tebben PJ, et al. Increasing incidence of nutritional rickets: a population-based study in Olmsted County, Minnesota. Mayo Clin Proc 2013;88(2):176–83.
30. Weisberg P, Scanlon KS, Li R, et al. Nutritional rickets among children in the United States: review of cases reported between 1986 and 2003. Am J Clin Nutr 2004;80(6 Suppl):1697S–705S.
31. Munns CF, Shaw N, Kiely M, et al. Global Consensus Recommendations on Prevention and Management of Nutritional Rickets. J Clin Endocrinol Metab 2016; 101(2):394–415.
32. Aung H, Soe K, Smithuis FF, et al. Case Report: Children with Severe Nutritional Rickets in the Naga Region in Northwest Myanmar, on the border with India. Am J Trop Med Hyg 2021;105(1):217–21.
33. Maiya S, Sullivan I, Allgrove J, et al. Hypocalcaemia and vitamin D deficiency: an important, but preventable, cause of life-threatening infant heart failure. Heart 2008;94(5):581–4.
34. Brooke OG, Brown IR, Bone CD, et al. Vitamin D supplements in pregnant Asian women: effects on calcium status and fetal growth. Br Med J 1980;280(6216): 751–4.
35. Iyer P, Diamond FB Jr. Shedding light on hypovitaminosis D and rickets. Adv Pediatr 2007;54:115–33.
36. Thoma ME, Drew LB, Hirai AH, et al. Black-White Disparities in Preterm Birth: Geographic, Social, and Health Determinants. Am J Prev Med 2019;57(5): 675–86.
37. Manuck TA. Racial and ethnic differences in preterm birth: A complex, multifactorial problem. Semin Perinatol 2017;41(8):511–8.
38. Bartick MC, Schwarz EB, Green BD, et al. Suboptimal breastfeeding in the United States: Maternal and pediatric health outcomes and costs. Matern Child Nutr 2017;13(1). https://doi.org/10.1111/mcn.12366.
39. Baker P, Smith JP, Garde A, et al. The political economy of infant and young child feeding: confronting corporate power, overcoming structural barriers, and accelerating progress. Lancet 2023;401(10375):503–24.
40. Perez-Escamilla R, Tomori C, Hernandez-Cordero S, et al. Breastfeeding: crucially important, but increasingly challenged in a market-driven world. Lancet 2023;401(10375):472–85.
41. Gartner LM, Greer FR. Section on B, Committee on Nutrition. American Academy of P. Prevention of rickets and vitamin D deficiency: new guidelines for vitamin D intake. Pediatrics 2003;111(4 Pt 1):908–10.
42. Lemoine A, Giabicani E, Lockhart V, et al. Case report of nutritional rickets in an infant following a vegan diet. Arch Pediatr 2020;27(4):219–22.
43. Martinez-Biarge M, Gould S, Alcalde de Alvare AD, et al. Lack of supplementation, and not a vegan diet, as a cause of rickets in an infant. Arch Pediatr 2021;28(3):255–6.
44. Iyer P, Diamond F. Detecting disorders of vitamin D deficiency in children: an update. Adv Pediatr 2013;60(1):89–106.
45. Ultraviolet light: a hazard to children. American Academy of Pediatrics. Committee on Environmental Health. Pediatrics 1999;104(2 Pt 1):328–33.
46. Blanco E, Burrows R, Reyes M, et al. Breastfeeding as the sole source of milk for 6 months and adolescent bone mineral density. Osteoporos Int 2017;28(10): 2823–30.

47. Carter SA, Parsons CM, Robinson SM, et al. Infant milk feeding and bone health in later life: findings from the Hertfordshire cohort study. Osteoporos Int 2020;31(4):709–14.
48. Uday S, Fratzl-Zelman N, Roschger P, et al. Cardiac, bone and growth plate manifestations in hypocalcemic infants: revealing the hidden body of the vitamin D deficiency iceberg. BMC Pediatr 2018;18(1):183.
49. Seymen-Karabulut G, Gunlemez A, Gokalp AS, et al. Vitamin D Deficiency Prevalence in Late Neonatal Hypocalcemia: A Multicenter Study. J Clin Res Pediatr Endocrinol 2021;13(4):384–90.
50. Do HJ, Park JS, Seo JH, et al. Neonatal Late-onset Hypocalcemia: Is There Any Relationship with Maternal Hypovitaminosis D? Pediatr Gastroenterol Hepatol Nutr 2014;17(1):47–51.
51. Khalesi N, Bahaeddini SM, Shariat M. Prevalence of maternal vitamin D deficiency in neonates with delayed hypocalcaemia. Acta Med Iran 2012;50(11):740–5.
52. Simon AE, Ahrens KA. Adherence to Vitamin D Intake Guidelines in the United States. Pediatrics 2020;145(6). https://doi.org/10.1542/peds.2019-3574.
53. Uday S, Kongjonaj A, Aguiar M, et al. Variations in infant and childhood vitamin D supplementation programmes across Europe and factors influencing adherence. Endocr Connect 2017;6(8):667–75.
54. Heaney RP. Calcium, dairy products and osteoporosis. J Am Coll Nutr 2000;19(2 Suppl):83S–99S.
55. Cormick G, Betran AP, Metz F, et al. Regulatory and Policy-Related Aspects of Calcium Fortification of Foods. Implications for Implementing National Strategies of Calcium Fortification. Nutrients 2020;12(4). https://doi.org/10.3390/nu12041022.
56. Cormick G, Betran AP, Romero IB, et al. Global inequities in dietary calcium intake during pregnancy: a systematic review and meta-analysis. BJOG 2019;126(4):444–56.
57. Malek AM, Newman JC, Hunt KJ, et al. Race/Ethnicity, Enrichment/Fortification, and Dietary Supplementation in the U.S. Population, NHANES 2009(-)2012. Nutrients 2019;11(5). https://doi.org/10.3390/nu11051005.
58. Pettifor JM, Ross P, Wang J, et al. Rickets in children of rural origin in South Africa: is low dietary calcium a factor? J Pediatr 1978;92(2):320–4.
59. Oginni LM, Sharp CA, Worsfold M, et al. Healing of rickets after calcium supplementation. Lancet 1999;353(9149):296–7.
60. Thacher TD, Fischer PR, Pettifor JM, et al. A comparison of calcium, vitamin D, or both for nutritional rickets in Nigerian children. N Engl J Med 1999;341(8):563–8.
61. Rana ZH, Bourassa MW, Gomes F, et al. Calcium status assessment at the population level: Candidate approaches and challenges. Ann N Y Acad Sci 2022;1517(1):93–106.
62. Silanikove N, Leitner G, Merin U. The Interrelationships between Lactose Intolerance and the Modern Dairy Industry: Global Perspectives in Evolutional and Historical Backgrounds. Nutrients 2015;7(9):7312–31.
63. Wang Y, Li S. Worldwide trends in dairy production and consumption and calcium intake: is promoting consumption of dairy products a sustainable solution for inadequate calcium intake? Food Nutr Bull 2008;29(3):172–85.
64. Eyberg CJ, Pettifor JM, Moodley G. Dietary calcium intake in rural black South African children. The relationship between calcium intake and calcium nutritional status. Hum Nutr Clin Nutr 1986;40(1):69–74.

65. Murphy SP, Beaton GH, Calloway DH. Estimated mineral intakes of toddlers: predicted prevalence of inadequacy in village populations in Egypt, Kenya, and Mexico. Am J Clin Nutr 1992;56(3):565–72.
66. Prentice A. Calcium intakes and bone densities of lactating women and breast-fed infants in The Gambia. Adv Exp Med Biol 1994;352:243–55.
67. Thacher TD, Fischer PR, Pettifor JM, et al. Case-control study of factors associated with nutritional rickets in Nigerian children. J Pediatr 2000;137(3):367–73.
68. Khandare AL, Harikumar R, Sivakumar B. Severe bone deformities in young children from vitamin D deficiency and fluorosis in Bihar-India. Calcif Tissue Int 2005;76(6):412–8.
69. Teotia M, Teotia SP, Singh KP. Endemic chronic fluoride toxicity and dietary calcium deficiency interaction syndromes of metabolic bone disease and deformities in India: year 2000. Indian J Pediatr 1998;65(3):371–81.
70. Jablonski NG, Chaplin G. Human skin pigmentation, migration and disease susceptibility. Philos Trans R Soc Lond B Biol Sci 2012;367(1590):785–92.
71. Holick MF. Sunlight and vitamin D for bone health and prevention of autoimmune diseases, cancers, and cardiovascular disease. Am J Clin Nutr 2004;80(6 Suppl):1678S–88S.
72. Loyal J, Cameron A. Vitamin D in Children: Can We Do Better? Pediatrics 2020;145(6). https://doi.org/10.1542/peds.2020-0504.
73. Gallo S, Gahche J, Kitsantas P, et al. Vitamin D Intake and Meeting Recommendations Among Infants Participating in WIC Nationally. J Nutr Educ Behav 2022;54(6):499–509.
74. Crocker B, Green TJ, Barr SI, et al. Very high vitamin D supplementation rates among infants aged 2 months in Vancouver and Richmond, British Columbia, Canada. BMC Publ Health 2011;11:905.
75. Rodd C, Jean-Philippe S, Vanstone C, et al. Comparison of 2 vitamin D supplementation modalities in newborns: adherence and preference. Appl Physiol Nutr Metab 2011;36(3):414–8.
76. Oberhelman SS, Meekins ME, Fischer PR, et al. Maternal vitamin D supplementation to improve the vitamin D status of breast-fed infants: a randomized controlled trial. Mayo Clin Proc 2013;88(12):1378–87.
77. Roth DE, Abrams SA, Aloia J, et al. Global prevalence and disease burden of vitamin D deficiency: a roadmap for action in low- and middle-income countries. Ann N Y Acad Sci 2018;1430(1):44–79.
78. Backstrand JR. The history and future of food fortification in the United States: a public health perspective. Nutr Rev 2002;60(1):15–26.
79. Springmann M, Freund F. Options for reforming agricultural subsidies from health, climate, and economic perspectives. Nat Commun 2022;13(1):82.
80. Springmann M, Wiebe K, Mason-D'Croz D, et al. Health and nutritional aspects of sustainable diet strategies and their association with environmental impacts: a global modelling analysis with country-level detail. Lancet Planet Health 2018;2(10):e451–61.
81. Palacios C, Cormick G, Hofmeyr GJ, et al. Calcium-fortified foods in public health programs: considerations for implementation. Ann N Y Acad Sci 2021;1485(1):3–21.
82. Chibuzor MT, Graham-Kalio D, Osaji JO, et al. Vitamin D, calcium or a combination of vitamin D and calcium for the treatment of nutritional rickets in children. Cochrane Database Syst Rev 2020;4(4):CD012581.
83. Bouillon R, Antonio L. Nutritional rickets: Historic overview and plan for worldwide eradication. J Steroid Biochem Mol Biol 2020;198:105563.

Racial and Ethnic Disparities in Access to and Outcomes of Infertility Treatment and Assisted Reproductive Technology in the United States

Gabriela Beroukhim, MD*, David B. Seifer, MD

KEYWORDS

• Racial disparities • Ethnic disparities • In vitro fertilization (IVF)
• Intrauterine insemination (IUI) • Assisted reproductive technology (ART)
• ART access • ART outcomes

KEY POINTS

- Racial and ethnic disparities are prevalent and persistent in access to and outcomes of infertility treatment and assisted reproductive technology (ART).
- Limited evidence assessing disparities in outcomes of intrauterine insemination suggests lower pregnancy rates among American Indian and Asian women, and comparable pregnancy rates among Black, Hispanic, and White women.
- Numerous studies indicate that favorable outcomes from autologous in vitro fertilization cycles are significantly lower among Black, Hispanic, and Asian women compared to White women.
- Race is an independent predictor of live birth success from ART.
- Potential explanations for disparities in infertility and ART treatment outcomes include limited access or delay to care —whether owing to socioeconomic status, status of insurance coverage, cultural or religious discomfort with medically assisted reproduction, experienced and/or perceived bias, and racism—as well as biological factors, such as differences in overall health and/or disease risk burden.

INTRODUCTION

In the United States, 10% to 15% of couples are unable to conceive after 1 year of unprotected intercourse.[1] The advent and advances in assisted reproductive technologies (ARTs) have enabled individuals and couples otherwise unable to conceive with

Department of Obstetrics, Gynecology, and Reproductive Sciences, Yale School of Medicine, 333 Cedar Street, New Haven, CT 06510, USA
* Corresponding author.
E-mail address: gabrielaberoukhim@gmail.com

Endocrinol Metab Clin N Am 52 (2023) 659–675
https://doi.org/10.1016/j.ecl.2023.05.005
endo.theclinics.com
0889-8529/23/

conventional methods to overcome infertility and achieve pregnancy. Still, a substantial number of individuals with infertility remain untreated or undertreated.[2–4] According to a panel of experts in 2009, approximately 25% of the needs for ART in the United States population were being met.[5]

Epidemiologic studies indicate that infertility disproportionately affects the minority, non-White populace.[6–9] In several US population-based studies, Black women have twofold increased odds of infertility compared to non-Hispanic White (NHW) women after adjusting for factors including socioeconomic status, correlates of pregnancy intent, and risk factors for infertility such as age, smoking status, testosterone levels, fibroid presence, and ovarian volume.[7–9] Moreover, Hispanic, non-Hispanic other races, and American Indian/Alaska Native women also have significantly higher rates of infertility compared to NHW women.[8,10] Disparities in prevalence of infertility in the United States may be because of gaps in overall health, gynecologic and reproductive wellness (ie, preventative care measures [ie, access to and utilization of contraception, human papilloma virus vaccination, and pre-exposure prophylaxis], comorbid gynecologic conditions affecting fertility (ie, uterine fibroids [UFs] and pelvic infections), dissemination of information, access to care, and racism, manifesting as poorer quality of care for the non-White minorities.[11]

Despite higher rates of infertility among non-White women, a disproportionately lower percentage of Black, Hispanic, non-Hispanic other races, American Indians, Alaska Natives, Native Hawaiians, or other Pacific Islanders, access and utilize fertility care compared with NHW women.[12] Black women specifically are half as likely to report having sought or accessed fertility treatment.[7,10,13,14] and are hugely underrepresented among those undergoing ART.[15] In an analysis of the National Survey of Family Growth (NSFG) database from 2002, 2006, to 2010, NHW women report receiving medical fertility assistance at nearly double the rates of non-White women.[16] Several other analyses of the NSFG database confirmed that Black and Hispanic women were significantly less likely than NHW to undergo testing and receive treatment after infertility evaluation (infertility testing: 8%–13% vs 69%; infertility treatment 6% vs 81%).[8,9,17,18] Data from the National Health and Nutrition Examination Survey (NHANES), reflecting responses from an estimated population of 45,576,559 US women, also revealed that Black and Mexican American women sought infertility care less frequently than Asian or NHW women (40%–44% vs 65%–80%, $P < 0.001$).[19] In a retrospective cohort study of US birth data files from 2011 to 2019, Black and Hispanic women were approximately 70% less likely to receive infertility treatment compared with NHW women.[20] Moreover, numerous studies indicate that Black, Hispanic, and Asian women tend to wait 20 to 24 months longer before seeking or accessing treatment of infertility compared with NHW women.[14,21–25] Likely owing to a delay in access to care, Black women tend to be older and have lower ovarian reserve indices (higher rates of diminished ovarian reserve (DOR) and lower age-matched serum anti-Mullerian hormone) compared with NHW women at the time of infertility treatment (**Fig. 1**).[6,26,27]

Even among individuals and couples who successfully access fertility care, disparities exist in the outcomes of treatment (ie, intrauterine insemination [IUI], ovulation induction, and in vitro fertilization [IVF]). Mounting evidence suggests that Black, Hispanic, and Asian women experience less favorable treatment outcomes than NHW women.[28] Because utilization of medically assisted reproduction is expected to continue to increase, the need to address and correct disparities in access to and outcomes of ART is even more relevant. In this review, we examine racial and ethnic disparities in outcomes of infertility treatment and ART for reproductive age women and couples in the United States. We also aim to explore the underpinnings of racial and

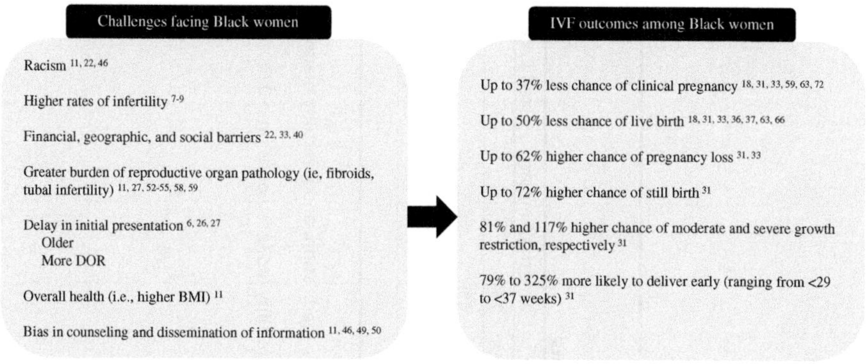

Fig. 1. Challenges contributing to disparities in outcomes of IVF among Black compared with White women.

ethnic disparities in fertility care and propose methods to provide possible solutions toward achieving improved equity.

Racial and Ethnic Disparities in Intrauterine Insemination Outcomes

Limited research lends insight into racial and ethnic disparities in outcomes of IUI (**Table 1**). In a retrospective analysis of 663 women, American Indian women undergoing IUI had significantly lower pregnancy rates (risk ratio [RR] 0.34, 95% confidence interval [CI] 0.16–0.72) and ongoing pregnancy/delivery rates (RR 0.33, 95% CI 0.12–0.87) when compared with NHW women, after controlling for cycle characteristics.[29] IUI outcomes for Black, Asian, and Hispanic women were comparable to NHW patients.[29] In a retrospective cohort study of 4,537 IUI cycles, there was no significant difference by race or ethnicity in rates of spontaneous abortion or clinical and multiple pregnancy rates.[24] In a retrospective cohort analysis of 814 Asian and NHW patients undergoing 2,327 IUI cycles, Asian women had significantly lower odds of pregnancy after adjusting for age, stimulation protocol, gravity and parity, and duration of infertility (adjusted odds ratio [aOR] 0.68, 95% CI 0.47–0.98, $P = 0.039$).[25]

Racial and Ethnic Disparities in Assisted Reproductive Technology/In Vitro Fertilization Treatment Outcomes

Ovarian response

Little data lend insight into disparities in oocyte yield following ovarian stimulation. In a Society for Assisted Reproductive Technologies Clinical Outcomes Reporting System (SART CORS) database analysis of 122,721 autologous, fresh, non-donor embryo cycles, Black women were significantly older, had higher rates of DOR (27.4% vs 21.5%; $P < 0.001$), had a lower mean number of oocytes retrieved (13.8 oocytes among NHB women vs 14.3 among White women, $P < 0.001$), and a higher cycle cancellation rate largely owing to poor ovarian response (12.9% vs 9.9%, $P < 0.001$).[27]

Clinical pregnancy rates

Consistent evidence indicates significant racial and ethnic differentials in rates of achieving clinical pregnancy (CP) with IVF (**Table 2**). A substantial amount of the data used to assess disparities in ART (DART) outcomes are derived from the SART CORS, a large, national, standardized IVF clinic-specific linked database that provides cumulative live birth (LB) rates from medically assisted reproduction in the United States.[30] In a SART CORS analysis of 225,889 autologous fresh embryo transfer cycles from 2004 to 2006, Black, Asian, and Hispanic women had significantly lower odds of

Table 1
Disparities in outcomes of intrauterine insemination by racial/ethnic group

Citation	Number of IUI Cycles	Outcome	Race/Ethnicity					
			NHW (Referent)	Black	Hispanic	Asian	American Indian	Mixed Race
Craig et al,[29] 2018	2,007	CPR	15.50%	11.60%	16.30%	16.70%	7%[a]	—
		Ongoing pregnancy/ delivery rate	10.50%	8.10%	9.80%	11.70%	4%	—
Dimitriadis et al,[24] 2017	4,537	CPR	11.90%	15%	13.80%	11.90%	—	11.50%
Lamb et al,[25] 2009	2,327	CPR	9.30%	—	—	7.1%[b]	—	—

Abbreviation: CPR, Clinical pregnancy rate.

[a] Statistical significance after adjusting for total motile sperm count, female age, body mass index, duration of infertility, medication, and infertility diagnosis (adjusted risk ratio 0.34, 95% CI 0.16–0.72).

[b] Statistical significance after adjusting for age, stimulation protocol, differences in gravity and parity, and duration of infertility (adjusted odds ratio 0.68, 95% CI 0.47–0.98).

Table 2
Disparities in outcomes of autologous in vitro fertilization cycles by racial/ethnic group

Citation	Number of IVF Cycles	Outcome	Race/Ethnicity		
			Black	Hispanic	Asian
Baker et al,[31] 2010	225,889 fresh cycles	CPR	↓	↓	↓
		LBR	↓↓	↓	↓
Fujimoto et al,[32] 2010	139,027 cycles	CPR	0	0	↓
		LBR	↓↓	↓	↓
Seifer et al,[15] 2008	61,575 fresh cycles	CPR	↓	—	—
		LBR	↓	—	—
	10,697 frozen cycles	CPR	0	—	—
		LBR	0	—	—
Seifer et al,[69] 2010	131,348 fresh cycles	CPR	↓	—	—
		LBR	↓	—	—
	27,345 frozen cycles	CPR	0	—	—
		LBR	0	—	—
Seifer et al,[27] 2020	122,721 fresh cycles	LBR	↓↓	—	—
Kotlyar et al,[35] 2021	148,572 fresh cycles	LBR	—	↓	↓
Sharara and McClamrock[79] 2000	168 cycles	CPR	↓↓	—	—
		LBR	↓↓	—	—
McCarthy-Keith et al,[73] 2010	2,050 fresh cycles	CPR	↓	↓	—
		LBR	↓	↓	—
Csokmay et al,[80] 2011	169 frozen cycles	CPR	0	—	—
		LBR	0	—	—
	98 fresh IVF transfers	CPR	0	—	—
		LBR	↓↓	—	—
Feinberg et al,[81] 2006	1,457 fresh cycles	CPR	0	0	—
		LBR	0	0	—
McQueen et al,[33] 2015	4,045 cycles	CPR	↓↓	0	↓
		LBR	↓↓	0	↓↓
Mascarenhas et al,[36] 2019	7,061 initial fresh transfers	LBR	↓↓	—	↓↓
	1,722 initial frozen transfers	LBR	0	—	0
Gleicher et al,[82] 2011	339 cycles	CPR	↓↓	—	—
Dayal et al,[83] 2009	251 initial fresh cycles	CPR	0	—	—
		LBR	0	—	—
Nichols et al,[84] 2001	358 fresh cycles	CPR	↑↑	—	—
Bendikson et al,[85] 2005	1,135 first cycles	LBR	0	0	0
Csokmay et al,[80] 2011	169 frozen cycles	CPR	0	—	—
		LBR	0	—	—
	98 fresh cycles	CPR	0		
		LBR	↓↓		
Rudik et al,[86] 2012	188 cycles	CPR	—	↓	↓
		LBR	—	↓	↓
Shuler et al,[87] 2011	435 initial fresh cycles	CPR	—	0	—
		LBR	—	0	—
Purcell et al,[37] 2007	27,272 cycles	CPR	—	—	↓
		LBR	—	—	↓
Kan et al,[88] 2015	2,594 cycles	CPR	—	—	0
		LBR	—	—	0

(*continued on next page*)

Table 2
(*continued*)

Citation	Number of IVF Cycles	Outcome	Race/Ethnicity		
Shahine et al,[89] 2009	225 cycles	CPR	—	—	↓↓
		LBR	—	—	↓↓
Palep-Singh et al,[90] 2007	608 fresh cycles	CPR	—	—	↓
		LBR	—	—	↓
Mahmud et al,[91] 1995	132 initial cycles	CPR	—	—	0
		LBR	—	—	0
Lashen et al,[92] 1999	324 cycles	CPR	—	—	0
Langen et al,[38] 2010	180 fresh transfers	CPR	—	—	↓
		LBR	—	—	↓

NHW as referent race.
Abbreviations: LBR, live birth rate; 0, no significant difference.

CP compared with NHWs.[31] In another SART CORS analysis of 139,027 ART cycles from 2004 to 2006, the odds of CP were significantly lower for Asians compared with NHWs (OR 0.86, 95% CI 0.80–0.93).[32] Among 4,045 women who underwent a first autologous IVF cycle in a single fertility center, CP was significantly lower among Black women (aOR = 0.63, 95% CI 0.44–0.88) and Asian women (aOR = 0.73, 95% CI 0.60–0.90) compared with NHW women, though not for Hispanic women.[33]

Live birth rates

Non-White women undergoing IVF also tend to have significantly lower LB rates (see **Table 2**). In a SART CORS analysis of 139,027 ART cycles from 2004 to 2006, the odds of LB were lower for Black (OR 0.62, 95% CI 0.56–0.68), Hispanic (OR 0.87, 95% CI 0.79–0.96), and Asian (OR 0.90, 95% CI 0.82–0.97) women compared with NHWs, after adjusting for maternal age, number of embryos transferred, and diagnoses of male factor, endometriosis, polycystic ovarian syndrome, DOR, tubal factor, uterine factor, and other factors.[32] In an analysis of SART CORS data from 1999, 2000, 2004, and 2008, among >120,000 IVF cycles, clinical intrauterine pregnancy and overall LB rates were lower among Black and Asian women.[15,33,34] Specifically, among 80,309 IVF cycles in 1999 and 2000, the LB rate was 26.3% among NHW women compared with 18.7% among Black women (rate ratio, 1.41).[15] After controlling for factors including increased tubal and uterine factor infertility among Black women, Black race was an independent risk factor for not achieving a LB (adjusted relative risk, 1.21; 95% CI, 1.12–1.36 if no prior ART, and RR, 1.38; 95% CI, 1.20–1.57 if prior ART).[15] Race remained an independent predictor of LB outcomes in an analysis of >100,000 fresh, autologous cycles between 2014 and 2016: Black, Hispanic, and Asian women had significantly lower LB rates and cumulative LB rates than NHW women, independent of factors such as age, parity, BMI, etiology of infertility, ovarian reserve, cycle cancellation, past spontaneous abortions, use of intracytoplasmic sperm injection, or number of embryos transferred.[27,35] Among women who underwent an initial autologous IVF, the OR for LB was 0.50 (95% CI 0.33–0.72) in Black women, 0.64 (95% CI 0.51–0.80) in Asian women, and 0.80 (95% CI 0.60–1.06) in Hispanic women compared with NHW women after adjusting for age, BMI, follicle stimulating hormone, smoking, and primary infertility diagnosis.[33] In a retrospective cohort study from 2010 to 2016, South Asian (aOR 0.62, 95% CI 0.53–0.73) and Black Afro-Caribbean women (aOR 0.53, 95% CI 0.33–0.84) had a lower LB rate per fresh embryo transfer compared with NHW women, though not for frozen embryo transfers.[36] In a SART analysis, Asian women had a decreased CP rate (OR = 0.71; 95% CI 0.64–0.80) and a decreased LB rate (OR = 0.69; 95% CI 0.61–0.77) compared with NHW women,[37] discrepancies that could not be accounted for by differences in age, infertility diagnosis (including DOR), parity, cycle day 3 FSH ratio, use of intracytoplasmic sperm injection, and number of embryos transferred.[37] In a retrospective review of 180 fresh blastocyst transfers from 2005 to 2006 among NHW and Asian women with comparable number of oocytes retrieved, fertilization rate, and number of blastocysts transferred, Asian women had a thicker endometrial lining yet a lower implantation rate (28% compared with 45%, $P = 0.01$), CP rate (43% compared with 59%, $P = 0.03$), and LB rate (31% compared with 48%, $P = 0.02$).[38] In multivariable analysis, the decreased LB rate among Asian women persisted (aOR = 0.48, 95% CI 0.24–0.96, $P = 0.004$).[38]

Among non-autologous embryo transfer cycles, those involving oocytes from Black donors (aRR 0.86, 95% CI 0.72, 1.03) and transfers to Black recipients (aRR 0.84, 95% CI 0.71, 0.99) had a lower probability of LB compared with NHW donors and NHW recipients, respectively.[39]

Pregnancy loss and neonatal mortality

Evidence suggests that non-White women undergoing IVF have significantly higher rates of pregnancy loss. In a SART CORS analysis of 225,889 autologous fresh embryo transfer cycles from 2004 to 2006, Hispanic and Asian women had a significantly greater risk of pregnancy loss in the second and third trimesters, and Black women had a significantly greater risk of pregnancy loss in all trimesters compared with NHWs ($aOR_{(\leq 8\ weeks)} = 0.83$, $P < 0.005$; $aOR_{(9\text{–}12\ weeks)} = 0.61$, $P < 0.0001$; $aOR_{(13\text{–}19\ weeks)} = 0.38$, $P < 0.0001$; $aOR_{(\geq 20\ weeks)} = 0.28$, $P < 0.0001$; $aOR_{(all\ weeks)} = 0.62$, $P < 0.0001$).[31] Among 4,045 first autologous IVF cycles, spontaneous abortion rates were 14.6% in NHW women versus 28.9% in Black women, 20.6% in Asian women, and 15.3% in Hispanic women.[33] In a SART-CORS analysis from 1999 to 2000 of 80,196 ART cycles, spontaneous abortion rates for fresh non-donor cycles with a clinical intrauterine gestation were significantly higher among Black women compared with NHW women, though comparable for cycles using cryopreserved embryos.[15,33,34]

In a population-based retrospective cohort study of 7,545,805 singleton births in the United States from 2016 to 2017, neonatal mortality was more than fourfold higher in infants of NHB women (aRR = 4.1, 95% CI 2.9–5.9) compared with NHW women conceiving using ART; this was in comparison to a nearly twofold higher risk (aRR = 1.9, 95% CI 1.8–1.9) for those conceiving spontaneously.[40]

Racial and Ethnic Disparities in Obstetrical Complications Following Assisted Reproductive Technology

Even once pregnancy is achieved, disparities persist in the obstetrical outcomes of pregnancies resulting from ART. In a SART CORS analysis of 139,027 ART, rates of moderate and severe growth restriction were increased for singleton infants among Asians (OR 1.78 and 2.05, respectively), Blacks (OR 1.81 and 2.17, respectively), and Hispanics (OR 1.36 and 1.64, respectively), compared with NHWs (see **Fig. 1**).[32] Black women were also 4.25 times as likely to deliver early (<29 weeks), 2.72 times as likely to deliver early (<32 weeks), and 1.79 times as likely to deliver preterm (<37 weeks), compared with NHW women; Hispanic women were 1.22 times more likely to deliver preterm (see **Fig. 1**).[32] Among twin pregnancies, the odds for moderate growth restriction were significantly increased for infants of Asian (OR 1.30) and Black women (OR 1.97), and severe growth restriction was increased among Black women (OR 3.21).[32]

Among pregnancies resulting naturally or from ART, non-White women experience higher rates of complications, including hypertensive disorders of pregnancy and gestational diabetes, diagnoses that are associated with yet other adverse pregnancy outcomes (ie, fetal demise, macrosomia, birth trauma, neonatal hypoglycemia) and have serious implications that outlast pregnancy (ie, higher risk of developing overt diabetes and cardiovascular disease).[41] In a 10 year longitudinal study among 2.5 million women, Black women had the highest rates of hypertensive disorders in pregnancy, including preeclampsia.[42] In a large NHANES study, Hispanic and Asian women had significantly higher rates of gestational diabetes, whereas Black women have significantly higher rates of pregestational diabetes compared with NHW women.[43] Black women also have a significantly higher risk of pregnancy-related morbidity and mortality.[44,45] According to the Centers for Disease Control and Prevention, pregnancy-related mortality between 2016 and 2018 among Black women was 41.4 per 100,000 live births, compared with 13.7 in NHW women.[46]

Factors contributing to racial and ethnic disparities in infertility treatment outcomes
Though evidence consistently demonstrates racial and ethnic disparities in access to as well as utilization of, and outcomes of ART, limited research lends insight into the factors contributing to such disparities. In the DART hypothesis proposed by Seifer and colleagues,[2] reasons for disparities in outcomes of ART are derived from some relative contribution of 4 general identified causes or challenges: (1) delay in obtaining treatment, (2) higher dropout during and following an unsuccessful ART treatment cycle, (3) provider factors, and (4) differences in patient biological factors (**Fig. 2**).

1. **Delay in obtaining treatment and higher dropout during and following unsuccessful ART treatment cycles**

Financial barriers to undergoing medically assisted reproduction, social influences, personal and cultural values, and structural factors, including racism, may all contribute to delays in access to care and higher rates of dicontinuation of care among women of color.[2,5] Among women evaluated for infertility, income and employment status are strongly correlated with the likelihood of seeking treatment.[17] Women of lower socioeconomic status are less likely to undergo infertility treatment despite having higher rates of infertility.[10,19] In addition to the high cost, undergoing ART often requires that individuals take time off from work to pursue treatment. Black and Hispanic women, particularly, are more likely to report having difficulty paying for and arranging work leave to undergo treatment.[22] Financial barriers may be compounded by geographic barriers, because an estimated 29% of reproductive-age women in the United States live in an area without ART clinics.[47]

Social and cultural influences may further alter perceptions of infertility and help-seeking behaviors.[48] For example, stigma or cultural discomfort with infertility labels and ART as well as an emphasis on privacy, may affect time to and utilization of fertility care.[25,49–52] In a NSFG study, marital status, education, and religion were among factors significantly associated with the likelihood of seeking an infertility evaluation.[17] Compared with NHW women, Hispanic, Asian, and Black women were up to 18 times more likely to be concerned about friends and family knowing about their infertility treatment.[22] Black women in particular reported the greatest concern regarding inability to conceive and disappointing their spouse (OR 3.8 and 4.3, respectively), whereas social stigmatization of infertility was of great concern to Asian-American women.[22] In-depth interviews revealed a recurring belief among Hispanic women that children were the basis of marital relationships and that childless marriages were considered failures,[49] feelings that may delay or avert treatment seeking.[48]

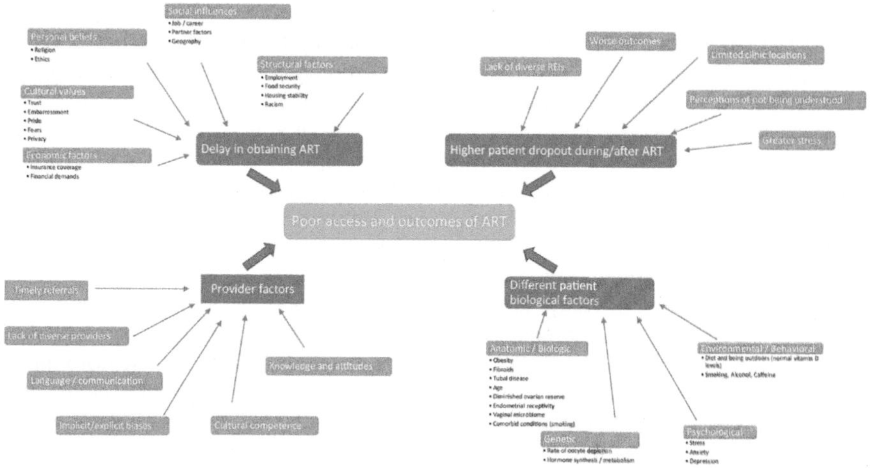

Fig. 2. The DART hypothesis of racial and ethnic disparities in access to and outcomes of IVF treatment in the United States. (*From* Seifer DB, Sharara FI, Jain T. The Disparities in ART (DART) Hypothesis of Racial and Ethnic Disparities in Access and Outcomes of IVF Treatment in the USA. Reprod Sci. 2022;29(7):2084-2088.)

Language differences may also impede access, which may be a challenge particularly relevant to immigrants or non-US citizens, who access infertility care significantly less compared with citizens.[19,50]

2. **Provider factors**

Implicit or explicit biases and racism are also recognized as plausible underpinnings of racial and ethnic disparities in fertility care.[11] In 27 in-depth interviews, women of color reported that some physicians dismiss their fertility concerns, assume they can get pregnant, emphasize birth control over procreation, and dissuade them from having children.[53] Hispanic and Black women, particularly, were more likely to report difficulty accessing treatment specifically because of race/ethnicity and acknowledge having difficulty scheduling an appointment and finding a physician with whom they thought comfortable.[22,54] Providers should also be sensitive to the reality that experienced and perceived racism, as well as the history of reproductive coercion, experimentation, and injustice, underlie medical mistrust among the collective memory of racial and ethnic minorities.[55,56] For example, Black women are 33 times more likely to be concerned about the historic misuse of medical treatment.[22] This is further reflected in the fivefold higher level of concern among Black women regarding the use of science to conceive.[22]

Provider bias in counseling may also be reflected in disparities in patient knowledge. Women from low resource, largely immigrant communities have greater disparities in fertility knowledge and lower health literacy compared with women from high-resource settings, despite comparable levels of education.[57] In a survey of over 400 women, non-White women had significantly lower awareness of risk factors for infertility, including smoking, obesity, and/or sexually transmitted infections, compared with NHW women.[58]

3. **Differences in patient biological factors**

Overall health, nutritional status, environmental exposures, housing quality, as well as physical, metabolic, and genetic confounders may contribute to the disparities in outcomes of medically assisted reproduction.[6,11] For example, higher exposure to endocrine disrupting chemicals commonly found in personal care products may be relevant to disparities in pregnancy outcomes.[59] During the prenatal period or pregnancy, phthalate metabolites and paraben concentrations were observed at higher levels in NHB and Hispanic women.[59] NHB women also reported higher usage of hair products, coinciding with a lower mean gestational age at deliver.[60] In another study, Hispanic women reported the highest total categories of personal care product usage in the first trimester, including use of hair products and perfume.[61] Possible biological factors contributing to racial and ethnic disparities in infertility treatment outcomes may include differentials in the vaginal microbiome, oocyte quality, embryo viability, endometrial factors, and hormonal milieu.[62]

Reproductive organ pathology tends to be higher among Black women and may contribute to poorer ART outcomes. Black women have up to a threefold greater incidence of UFs compared with NHW women, and are more likely to be symptomatic, have a larger volume of UFs, be offered a lesser spectrum of treatment options, and experience disparate treatment outcomes.[63–66] The greater UF burden affecting Black women may be consequent to racism leading to delays in access to and suboptimal treatment modalities available to Black, or biological differences, including the prevalence of vitamin D deficiency and certain genomic signals, such as mutations in mediator complex subunit 12, which are more common in Black women and are suggested to play a causative role in the pathogenesis of UFs.[67,68] Tubal factor infertility (TFI), a cause of infertility in nearly one-third of cases, also disproportionately affects Black women.[69] Black women affected by chlamydia are five times more likely than White women to develop TFI, which has largely been attributed to insufficient screening, treatment, and barriers in access to care for STI prevention and treatment.[11,70] Among women undergoing ART, Black women were found to have a significantly higher frequency of hydrosalpinx compared with NHW women, potentially contributing to a less receptive endometrium and reduced implantation.[27]

Potential mitigating factors

Collaborative efforts are necessary to critically assess the underpinnings of the racial and ethnic disparities in access, treatment, and outcomes of ART and to strategize towards attaining of equity in fertility care in the United States.[71] Professional organizations, academic institutions, and government-sponsored agencies will need to further continue to prioritize disparity-focused research and advocacy. Other measures that could be undertaken by government agencies entail improving access to preventative reproductive health care and infertility treatments through modifications in policies and politics. For example, expansion of Medicaid programs in Michigan has been associated with a reported improvement to access to birth control and family planning services,[72] underscoring the importance of Medicaid expansion for achieving improved and equitable access to reproductive care. Moreover, directed efforts to address economic barriers in access to fertility care through enhanced or equal access to care models (eg, states that mandate third party-payer coverage of ART and military populations) may to some degree mitigate disparities in access to fertility care. A sensitivity analysis of SART-CORS data in mandated states indicated that the proportion of ART cycles among Black women was representative of the Black population, and Black women undergoing ART saw significantly higher LB rates compared with ART outcomes in non-mandated states.[27] In military ART programs, utilization of ART services by Black women was nearly fourfold higher than US ART demographic data, though significant disparities persisted in treatment outcomes.[73] Although equal access models are valuable, they are not sufficient to overcome DART. Despite state law-mandated insurance coverage of ART in 10 states, IVF services continue to be primarily accessed by highly educated, wealthy, NHW women.[74] Two well-designed studies examined the issue of how state-mandated insurance impacts racial/ethnic disparities in access to and outcomes in IVF using the SART-CORS database: (1) in an analysis of autologous IVF cycles from 2014 to 2019, state health insurance mandates did not mitigate racial and ethnic disparities in utilization of IVF and clinical outcomes,[75] (2) in an analysis of donor egg IVF cycles from 2014 to 2016, state health insurance mandates did not resolve racial and ethnic disparities in clinical outcomes.[76] In another example, enhanced access in military settings also did not attenuate disparities in access and utilization of fertility services for Hispanic individuals, who remain significantly underrepresented in ART use.[73,77] In Massachusetts, a state mandating coverage for infertility procedures as well as oocyte cryopreservation without individual requirements, limitations, or an annual/lifetime cap on coverage, Hispanic women remain underrepresented among utilizers of ART services.[74] Similarly, in Chicago, Illinois, where Blacks make up approximately 30% of the population, only 5.3% of Black women received treatment of infertility at Fertility Centers of Illinois, despite state-mandated infertility treatment coverage.[33] This underrepresentation of Black and Hispanic women may in part be because of a lack of awareness of insurance benefits. Black and Hispanic women in Illinois were approximately twice as likely to report income level as a barrier to fertility testing and treatment compared with NHW and Asian respondents.[54] In a cross-sectional survey among reproductive age women in Boston, Massachusetts, cost was the most reported barrier to care regardless of race/ethnicity, or insurance status, and only 8.9% of participants were aware of personal insurance coverage for infertility treatment.[78] Hispanic patients were less likely than NHW patients to know if their own insurance covered infertility treatment after adjusting for a personal history of infertility.[78] Persistent disparities in insurance-mandated states may also be because mandates only serve a subset of the population with employer-sponsored private insurance, thus excluding uninsured patients and beneficiaries of Medicaid.

Other potential mitigating factors include improving patient experiences and patient–provider interactions. Providers must reflect upon, address, and overcome race-based and class-based assumptions. In addition, broadening representation in the health care workforce can minimize patient and provider discordance, enhance cultural competency, maximize trust, and improve patient experiences. Efforts should be made to improve awareness among providers, patients, and their partners to understand the relevance of the biological clock and earlier access for better age-related outcomes. Referral to a specialist in reproductive medicine should be based on the age-specific recommendations of the American Society of Reproductive Medicine. Women less than 35 should be referred at 1 year after having unprotected intercourse whereas only after 6 months if age 35 or older, and if greater than 40, referral should be immediate to avoid exacerbation of age-related infertility. Further efforts to destigmatize infertility as a personal impairment and to encourage it to be viewed as a treatable disease will hopefully encourage more women of color to seek timely infertility care.

SUMMARY

Racial and ethnic disparities in infertility treatment and ART have been and continue to be conspicuously present. Numerous robust studies reveal significantly less favorable CP rates, LB rates with greater pregnancy loss, fetal growth restriction, and preterm birth rates among Black, Asian, and Hispanic women following IVF. However, several limitations are notable in the data. Large national databases, such as SART CORS, have approximately 35% of cycles of unknown race and ethnicity, qualifying the conclusions that may be surmised from such studies.[75] Other considerations include the imperfect methodological features of the cited survey studies, which can be subjected to response and recall bias.

To address such disparities and attain equity and equality in the desired family building, greater efforts will need to continue to be made to recognize and challenge racial and ethnic disparities. Efforts should be multipronged and systematic, aimed at eliminating discriminatory practices in reproductive medicine, delivering accurate, unbiased, culturally sensitive reproductive education, optimizing access to and quality of preventative reproductive care, addressing the comorbidities of women of color, destigmatizing infertility, and achieving timely access to infertility care for all. To identify other spaces where efforts should be focused, future studies could consider accounting for confounding social factors such as socioeconomic and insurance status, as well as exploring the partner's attitude, which may contribute to disparities.

CLINICS CARE POINTS

- Providers should be mindful of factors perpetuating disparities in access and utilization of infertility care, including racism, cultural and societal pressures, and cost. Providers should recognize barriers to infertility care and advocate for accessible and affordable treatment.
- Race/ethnicity, like age and BMI, is an independent predictor of LB success in ART. Providers should be aware of other contributing factors (ie, more likely to have delayed presentation to a specialist in reproductive medicine, being older, higher BMI, and having tubal and uterine pathology) to lower favorable outcomes of IVF among Black, Asian, and Hispanic women.
- Referral to a specialist in reproductive medicine should be expeditious and based on age-specific recommendations: (1) women less than age 35 should be referred one year after having unprotected intercourse, (2) women aged 35 to 39 should be referred after 6 months, and (3) women greater than age 40 should be referred immediately to avoid exacerbation of age-related infertility. Both referring physicians and their patients should be aware of these age-specific recommendations.

DISCLOSURE

The authors have no conflicts of interest to disclose.

REFERENCES

1. Practice Committee of the American Society for Reproductive M, the Practice Committee of the Society for Reproductive E, Infertility. Electronic address aao. Optimizing natural fertility: a committee opinion. Fertil Steril 2022;117(1):53–63.
2. Seifer DB, Sharara FI, Jain T. The Disparities in ART (DART) Hypothesis of Racial and Ethnic Disparities in Access and Outcomes of IVF Treatment in the USA. Reprod Sci 2022;29(7):2084–8.
3. Jain T, Harlow BL, Hornstein MD. Insurance coverage and outcomes of in vitro fertilization. N Engl J Med 2002;347(9):661–6.
4. Jackson-Bey TMJ, Jasper E, Edwards DRV, et al. Systematic review of racial and ethnic disparities in reproductive endocrinology and infertility: where do we stand today? Fertil Steril 2021;2(1):169–88.
5. Chambers GM, Sullivan EA, Ishihara O, et al. The economic impact of assisted reproductive technology: a review of selected developed countries. Fertil Steril 2009;91(6):2281–94.

6. Quinn M, Fujimoto V. Racial and ethnic disparities in assisted reproductive technology access and outcomes. Fertil Steril 2016;105(5):1119–23.
7. Wellons MF, Lewis CE, Schwartz SM, et al. Racial differences in self-reported infertility and risk factors for infertility in a cohort of black and white women: the CARDIA Women's Study. Fertil Steril 2008;90(5):1640–8.
8. Craig LB, Peck JD, Janitz AE. The prevalence of infertility in American Indian/Alaska Natives and other racial/ethnic groups: National Survey of Family Growth. Paediatr Perinat Epidemiol 2019;33(2):119–25.
9. Chandra A, Copen CE, Stephen EH. Infertility service use in the United States: data from the National Survey of Family Growth, 1982-2010. Natl Health Stat Report 2014;(73):1–21.
10. Bitler M, Schmidt L. Health disparities and infertility: impacts of state-level insurance mandates. Fertil Steril 2006;85(4):858–65.
11. Beroukhim G, Mahabamunuge J, Pal L. Racial disparities in access to reproductive health and fertility care in the United States. Curr Opin Obstet Gynecol 2022; 34(3):138–46.
12. Ebeh DN, Jahanfar S. Association between maternal race and the use of assisted reproductive technology in the USA. SN Compr Clin Med 2021;3(5):1106–14.
13. Ekechi C. Addressing inequality in fertility treatment. Lancet 2021;398(10301): 645–6.
14. Chin HB, Howards PP, Kramer MR, et al. Racial disparities in seeking care for help getting pregnant. Paediatr Perinat Epidemiol 2015;29(5):416–25.
15. Seifer DB, Frazier LM, Grainger DA. Disparity in assisted reproductive technologies outcomes in black women compared with white women. Fertil Steril 2008; 90(5):1701–10.
16. Blanchfield BV, Patterson CJ. Racial and sexual minority women's receipt of medical assistance to become pregnant. Health Psychol 2015;34(6):571–9.
17. Kessler LM, Craig BM, Plosker SM, et al. Infertility evaluation and treatment among women in the United States. Fertil Steril 2013;100(4):1025–32.
18. Janitz AE, Peck JD, Craig LB. Racial/Ethnic differences in the utilization of infertility services: a focus on American indian/alaska natives. Matern Child Health J 2019;23(1):10–8.
19. Kelley AS, Qin Y, Marsh EE, et al. Disparities in accessing infertility care in the United States: results from the National Health and Nutrition Examination Survey, 2013-16. Fertil Steril 2019;112(3):562–8.
20. Dongarwar D, Mercado-Evans V, Adu-Gyamfi S, et al. Racial/ethnic disparities in infertility treatment utilization in the US, 2011-2019. Syst Biol Reprod Med 2022; 68(3):180–9.
21. Jain T. Socioeconomic and racial disparities among infertility patients seeking care. Fertil Steril 2006;85(4):876–81.
22. Missmer SA, Seifer DB, Jain T. Cultural factors contributing to health care disparities among patients with infertility in Midwestern United States. Fertil Steril 2011; 95(6):1943–9.
23. Armstrong A, Plowden TC. Ethnicity and assisted reproductive technologies. Clin Pract (Lond) 2012;9(6):651–8.
24. Dimitriadis I, Batsis M, Petrozza JC, et al. Racial disparities in fertility care: an analysis of 4537 intrauterine insemination cycles. J Racial Ethn Health Disparities 2017;4(2):169–77.
25. Lamb JD, Huddleston HG, Purcell KJ, et al. Asian ethnicity is associated with decreased pregnancy rates following intrauterine insemination. Reprod Biomed Online 2009;19(2):252–6.

26. Seifer DB, Golub ET, Lambert-Messerlian G, et al. Variations in serum mullerian inhibiting substance between white, black, and Hispanic women. Fertil Steril 2009;92(5):1674–8.
27. Seifer DB, Simsek B, Wantman E, et al. Status of racial disparities between black and white women undergoing assisted reproductive technology in the US. Reprod Biol Endocrinol 2020;18(1):113.
28. Humphries LA, Chang O, Humm K, et al. Influence of race and ethnicity on in vitro fertilization outcomes: systematic review. Am J Obstet Gynecol 2016;214(2):212 e211–e212 e217.
29. Craig LB, Weedin EA, Walker WD, et al. Racial and ethnic differences in pregnancy rates following intrauterine insemination with a focus on American indians. J Racial Ethn Health Disparities 2018;5(5):1077–83.
30. Curchoe CL, Tarafdar O, Aquilina MC, et al. SART CORS IVF registry: looking to the past to shape future perspectives. J Assist Reprod Genet 2022;39(11):2607–16.
31. Baker VL, Luke B, Brown MB, et al. Multivariate analysis of factors affecting probability of pregnancy and live birth with in vitro fertilization: an analysis of the Society for Assisted Reproductive Technology Clinic Outcomes Reporting System. Fertil Steril 2010;94(4):1410–6.
32. Fujimoto VY, Luke B, Brown MB, et al. Racial and ethnic disparities in assisted reproductive technology outcomes in the United States. Fertil Steril 2010;93(2):382–90.
33. McQueen DB, Schufreider A, Lee SM, et al. Racial disparities in in vitro fertilization outcomes. Fertil Steril 2015;104(2):398–402 e391.
34. Grainger DS D, Frazier L, Rall M, et al. Racial disparity in clinical outcomes from women using advanced reproductive technologies (ART): analysis of 80,196 ART cycles from the SART database 1999 and 2000. Fertil Steril 2004;82:S37–8.
35. Kotlyar AM, Simsek B, Seifer DB. Disparities in ART live birth and cumulative live birth outcomes for hispanic and asian women compared to white non-hispanic women. J Clin Med 2021;10(12):2615.
36. Mascarenhas M, Balen AH. Could ethnicity have a different effect on fresh and frozen embryo transfer outcomes: a retrospective study. Reprod Biomed Online 2019;39(5):764–9.
37. Purcell K, Schembri M, Frazier LM, et al. Asian ethnicity is associated with reduced pregnancy outcomes after assisted reproductive technology. Fertil Steril 2007;87(2):297–302.
38. Langen ES, Shahine LK, Lamb JD, et al. Asian ethnicity and poor outcomes after in vitro fertilization blastocyst transfer. Obstet Gynecol 2010;115(3):591–6.
39. Liu Y, Hipp HS, Nagy ZP, et al. The effect of donor and recipient race on outcomes of assisted reproduction. Am J Obstet Gynecol 2021;224(4):374 e371–e374 e312.
40. Lisonkova S, Ukah UV, John S, et al. Racial and ethnic disparities in the perinatal health of infants conceived by ART. Pediatrics 2022;150(5). e2021055855.
41. Powe CE, Carter EB. Racial and ethnic differences in gestational diabetes: time to get serious. JAMA 2021;326(7):616–7.
42. Tanaka M, Jaamaa G, Kaiser M, et al. Racial disparity in hypertensive disorders of pregnancy in New York State: a 10-year longitudinal population-based study. Am J Public Health 2007;97(1):163–70.
43. Shah NS, Wang MC, Freaney PM, et al. Trends in gestational diabetes at first live birth by race and ethnicity in the US, 2011-2019. JAMA 2021;326(7):660–9.

44. Hoyert DL, Minino AM. Maternal mortality in the UNITED states: changes in coding, publication, and data release, 2018. Natl Vital Stat Rep 2020;69(2):1–18.
45. Hauspurg A, Lemon L, Cabrera C, et al. Racial differences in postpartum blood pressure trajectories among women after a hypertensive disorder of pregnancy. JAMA Netw Open 2020;3(12):e2030815.
46. Center for Disease Control and Prevention (CDC). Pregnancy Mortality Surveillance System. Available at: https://www.cdc.gov/reproductivehealth/maternal-mortality/pregnancy-mortality-surveillance-system.htm. Accessed May 1, 2023.
47. Harris JA, Menke MN, Haefner JK, et al. Geographic access to assisted reproductive technology health care in the United States: a population-based cross-sectional study. Fertil Steril 2017;107(4):1023–7.
48. White L, McQuillan J, Greil AL. Explaining disparities in treatment seeking: the case of infertility. Fertil Steril 2006;85(4):853–7.
49. Becker G, Castrillo M, Jackson R, et al. Infertility among low-income Latinos. Fertil Steril 2006;85(4):882–7.
50. Nachtigall RD, Castrillo M, Shah N, et al. The challenge of providing infertility services to a low-income immigrant Latino population. Fertil Steril 2009;92(1):116–23.
51. Inhorn MC, Fakih MH. Arab Americans, African Americans, and infertility: barriers to reproduction and medical care. Fertil Steril 2006;85(4):844–52.
52. Fujimoto VY, Jain T, Alvero R, et al. Proceedings from the conference on reproductive problems in women of color. Fertil Steril 2010;94(1):7–10.
53. Bell AV. Beyond (financial) accessibility: inequalities within the medicalisation of infertility. Sociol Health Illn 2010;32(4):631–46.
54. Galic I, Negris O, Warren C, et al. Disparities in access to fertility care: who's in and who's out. F S Rep 2021;2(1):109–17.
55. Rose A, Peters N, Shea JA, et al. Development and testing of the health care system distrust scale. J Gen Intern Med 2004;19(1):57–63.
56. Bogart LM, Bird ST, Walt LC, et al. Association of stereotypes about physicians to health care satisfaction, help-seeking behavior, and adherence to treatment. Soc Sci Med 2004;58(6):1049–58.
57. Hoffman JR, Delaney MA, Valdes CT, et al. Disparities in fertility knowledge among women from low and high resource settings presenting for fertility care in two United States metropolitan centers. Fertil Res Pract 2020;6:15.
58. Siegel DR, Sheeder J, Polotsky AJ. Racial and ethnic disparities in fertility awareness among reproductive-aged women. Womens Health Rep (New Rochelle) 2021;2(1):347–54.
59. Chan M, Mita C, Bellavia A, et al. Racial/ethnic disparities in pregnancy and prenatal exposure to endocrine-disrupting chemicals commonly used in personal care products. Curr Environ Health Rep 2021;8(2):98–112.
60. Preston EV, Fruh V, Quinn MR, et al. Endocrine disrupting chemical-associated hair product use during pregnancy and gestational age at delivery: a pilot study. Environ Health 2021;20(1):86.
61. Preston EV, Chan M, Nozhenko K, et al. Socioeconomic and racial/ethnic differences in use of endocrine-disrupting chemical-associated personal care product categories among pregnant women. Environ Res 2021;198:111212.
62. Aly J, Plowden TC, Christy AY. Factors contributing to persistent disparate outcomes of in vitro fertilization treatment. Curr Opin Obstet Gynecol 2021;33(4):335–42.
63. Wise LA, Laughlin-Tommaso SK. Epidemiology of uterine fibroids: from menarche to menopause. Clin Obstet Gynecol 2016;59(1):2–24.

64. Marsh EE, Ekpo GE, Cardozo ER, et al. Racial differences in fibroid prevalence and ultrasound findings in asymptomatic young women (18-30 years old): a pilot study. Fertil Steril 2013;99(7):1951–7.
65. Jacoby VL, Fujimoto VY, Giudice LC, et al. Racial and ethnic disparities in benign gynecologic conditions and associated surgeries. Am J Obstet Gynecol 2010; 202(6):514–21.
66. Eltoukhi HM, Modi MN, Weston M, et al. The health disparities of uterine fibroid tumors for African American women: a public health issue. Am J Obstet Gynecol 2014;210(3):194–9.
67. Baird DD, Hill MC, Schectman JM, et al. Vitamin d and the risk of uterine fibroids. Epidemiology 2013;24(3):447–53.
68. He C, Nelson W, Li H, et al. Frequency of MED12 mutation in relation to tumor and patient's clinical characteristics: a meta-analysis. Reprod Sci 2022;29(2):357–65.
69. Seifer DB, Zackula R, Grainger DA, Society for Assisted Reproductive Technology Writing Group R. Trends of racial disparities in assisted reproductive technology outcomes in black women compared with white women: Society for Assisted Reproductive Technology 1999 and 2000 vs. 2004-2006. Fertil Steril 2010;93(2): 626–35.
70. Chambers LC, Khosropour CM, Katz DA, et al. Racial/ethnic disparities in the lifetime risk of chlamydia trachomatis diagnosis and adverse reproductive health outcomes among women in king county, Washington. Clin Infect Dis 2018;67(4): 593–9.
71. Sutton MY, Anachebe NF, Lee R, et al. Racial and ethnic disparities in reproductive health services and outcomes, 2020. Obstet Gynecol 2021;137(2):225–33.
72. Moniz MH, Kirch MA, Solway E, et al. Association of access to family planning services with medicaid expansion among female enrollees in Michigan. JAMA Netw Open 2018;1(4):e181627.
73. McCarthy-Keith DM, Schisterman EF, Robinson RD, et al. Will decreasing assisted reproduction technology costs improve utilization and outcomes among minority women? Fertil Steril 2010;94(7):2587–9.
74. Jain T, Hornstein MD. Disparities in access to infertility services in a state with mandated insurance coverage. Fertil Steril 2005;84(1):221–3.
75. Correia KFB, Kraschel K, Seifer DB. State insurance mandates for in vitro fertilization are not associated with improving racial and ethnic disparities in utilization and treatment outcomes. Am J Obstet Gynecol 2023;(228). 313.e311-318.
76. Liao CKA, Seifer DB. Effect of state insurance mandates on racial/ethnic disparities in utilization and outcomes of donor oocyte assisted reproductive technologies. Fertil Steril 2023. https://doi.org/10.1016/j.fertnstert.2023.02.037.
77. Feinberg EC, Larsen FW, Wah RM, et al. Economics may not explain Hispanic underutilization of assisted reproductive technology services. Fertil Steril 2007; 88(5):1439–41.
78. Insogna IG, Lanes A, Hariton E, et al. Self-reported barriers to accessing infertility care: patient perspectives from urban gynecology clinics. J Assist Reprod Genet 2020;37(12):3007–14.
79. Sharara FI, McClamrock HD. Differences in in vitro fertilization (IVF) outcome between white and black women in an inner-city, university-based IVF program. Fertil Steril 2000;73(6):1170–3.
80. Csokmay JM, Hill MJ, Maguire M, et al. Are there ethnic differences in pregnancy rates in African-American versus white women undergoing frozen blastocyst transfers? Fertil Steril 2011;95(1):89–93.

81. Feinberg EC, Larsen FW, Catherino WH, et al. Comparison of assisted reproductive technology utilization and outcomes between Caucasian and African American patients in an equal-access-to-care setting. Fertil Steril 2006;85(4):888–94.
82. Gleicher N, Weghofer A, Lee IH, et al. Association of FMR1 genotypes with in vitro fertilization (IVF) outcomes based on ethnicity/race. PLoS One 2011;6(4):e18781.
83. Dayal MB, Gindoff P, Dubey A, et al. Does ethnicity influence in vitro fertilization (IVF) birth outcomes? Fertil Steril 2009;91(6):2414–8.
84. Nichols JE Jr, Higdon HL 3rd, Crane MMt, et al. Comparison of implantation and pregnancy rates in African American and white women in an assisted reproductive technology practice. Fertil Steril 2001;76(1):80–4.
85. Bendikson K, Cramer DW, Vitonis A, et al. Ethnic background and in vitro fertilization outcomes. Int J Gynaecol Obstet 2005;88(3):342–6.
86. Rudick B, Ingles S, Chung K, et al. Characterizing the influence of vitamin D levels on IVF outcomes. Hum Reprod 2012;27(11):3321–7.
87. Shuler A, Rodgers AK, Budrys NM, et al. In vitro fertilization outcomes in Hispanics versus non-Hispanic whites. Fertil Steril 2011;95(8):2735–7.
88. Kan A, Leung P, Luo K, et al. Do Asian women do as well as their Caucasian counterparts in IVF treatment: Cohort study. J Obstet Gynaecol Res 2015; 41(6):946–51.
89. Shahine LK, Lamb JD, Lathi RB, et al. Poor prognosis with in vitro fertilization in Indian women compared to Caucasian women despite similar embryo quality. PLoS One 2009;4(10):e7599.
90. Palep-Singh M, Picton HM, Vrotsou K, et al. South Asian women with polycystic ovary syndrome exhibit greater sensitivity to gonadotropin stimulation with reduced fertilization and ongoing pregnancy rates than their Caucasian counterparts. Eur J Obstet Gynecol Reprod Biol 2007;134(2):202–7.
91. Mahmud G, Lopez Bernal A, Yudkin P, et al. A controlled assessment of the in vitro fertilization performance of British women of Indian origin compared with white women. Fertil Steril 1995;64(1):103–6.
92. Lashen H, Afnan M, Sharif K. A controlled comparison of ovarian response to controlled stimulation in first generation Asian women compared with white Caucasians undergoing in vitro fertilisation. Br J Obstet Gynaecol 1999;106(5):407–9.

Challenges of Gender-Affirming Care in Incarcerated Transgender People

Rana Malek, MD[a,*], Mauro Sarmiento, MD, PhD[b], Elizabeth Lamos, MD[a]

KEYWORDS

• Health disparities • Health vulnerabilities • Incarceration • Transgender

KEY POINTS

- Transgender people are at higher risk for justice system involvement.
- The World Professional Association for Transgender Health (WPATH) Standards of Care-8 state that all institutionalized transgender individuals receive gender affirming care.
- Inconsistent legal policies and systemic barriers in the United States Correctional System result in variable gender-affirming care.
- Endocrinologists educated on the structural, interpersonal, and educational barriers to care can be empowered to navigate these complexities to improve the health of incarcerated transgender individuals.

INTRODUCTION

Social and health disparities among transgender people have been increasingly well described in the literature.[1–3] For transgender people, health vulnerabilities exist within a cycle. Transgender people face discrimination and challenges in the social determinants of health, including education, housing, and employment.[4] These challenges result in less access to societal safety nets and resources like reliable support systems and health care. Past negative experiences within the health care system have violated the trust of the transgender community. The stigma and discrimination that they face in health care settings manifest in health vulnerabilities such as high rates of smoking, diagnosis of HIV, psychological stress, concerning rates of suicide and suicide attempts, and inequitable preventative health care.[1,2,5–7]

In addition, transgender people experience alarming exposure to violence and assault.[1,2] Reports suggest increased interaction with police and law enforcement,

[a] University of Maryland School of Medicine, 800 Linden Avenue, 8th Floor UMCDE, Baltimore, MD 21201, USA; [b] YesCare Corporation, 7240 Parkway Drive, Suite 350, Hanover, MD 21076, USA
* Corresponding author.
E-mail address: rmalek@som.umaryland.edu

Endocrinol Metab Clin N Am 52 (2023) 677–687
https://doi.org/10.1016/j.ecl.2023.05.007
endo.theclinics.com
0889-8529/23/

particularly among Black transgender women. The challenges placed on incarcerated transgender people to receive gender-affirming care are amplified by the existing policies, bias, structure, and binary system of incarceration.[8] Incarcerated transgender people are a unique population, often overlooked, and this article will seek to highlight some of the challenges that they face.

The endocrinologist may participate in the care of a transgender person within a spectrum of social/societal circumstances, of which incarceration is one (**Fig. 1**).

At Risk of Incarceration

These individuals present to an endocrinology clinic seeking gender affirming care and upon a thorough medical and social history, the provider identifies potential factors correlating with incarceration. Several risk factors can be identified that may lead to more interaction with police, resulting in incarceration (**Table 1**).[2,9] These include a history of homelessness, current homelessness, prior incarceration, school dropout, and participation in illegal underground employment (sex work or selling drugs), for example, White Hughto and colleagues also reported that lifetime sexual, physical assault, or verbal harassment, being a transgender woman, living with HIV, and polysubstance use within the past year increased the odds of lifetime incarceration.[10] Addressing these concerns is outside the scope of this article, but there are opportunities to intervene with resources such as mental health care, case management, and social work to attempt to break the cycle of vulnerability.[9,11,12]

Currently Incarcerated

The scope of incarceration for transgender people is unclear. These data are limited and likely an underestimate given the use of self-reporting, the population sample, and the survey design.[13] In addition, federal and state institutions do not uniformly collect gender identity information for reporting purposes. For example, it was only in 2014 that the Bureau of Justice Statistics added transgender and intersex as gender categories for the Survey of Sexual Victimization.[14] In contrast, the recent report on Length of Incarceration and Recidivism (2022) from the US Sentencing Commission did not include gender identity.[15] Mistrust in the medical system and distrust of the

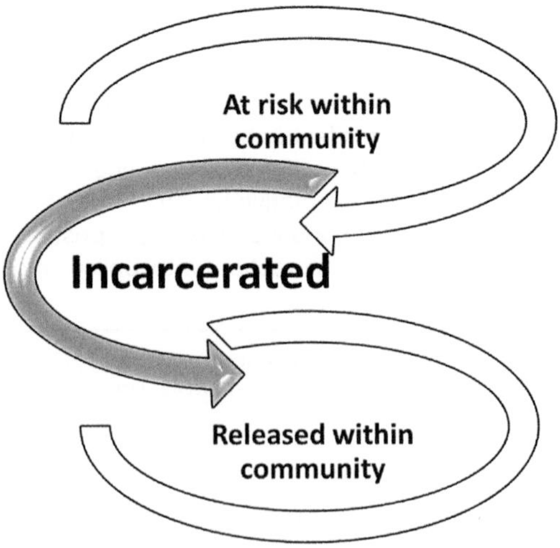

Fig. 1. Spectrum of incarceration.

Table 1
Social vulnerabilities reported by transgender people result in increased reports of incarceration

Social Vulnerability Reported by Individuals	Percent Reporting Incarceration at Some Point or for Any Reason	Comparison to Those Who Did Not Report Social Vulnerability
Physically assaulted in school	22%	N/A
Sexually assaulted in school	24%	N/A
Currently homeless	49%	15% (3x higher)
Domestic violence related to nonaccepting family	29%	11%
Family rejection	19%	11%
Sex work	48%	16%[a]
Unemployed	24%	13%
Lost job because of bias	24%	N/A
Experienced prior homelessness	34%	13% (2.5x increase)

Abbreviation: N/A, not available.
[a] Comparison to overall sample.
Data from Grant JMLTJHJHJKM. *Injustice at Every Turn. A Report of the National Transgender Discrimination Survey.*; 2011. https://transequality.org/sites/default/files/docs/resources/NTDS_Report.pdf.

corrections/police environment because of prior experiences and fear of harassment/information sharing may all contribute to underreporting of data.[1,2]

In a survey of 6,450 transgender and gender nonconforming individuals, 16% of respondents indicated that they were jailed in their lifetime, compared with 2.7% of the general US population.[2] Those who went to jail or prison disproportionately identified as Black, American Indian, or Latino as compared with White and were more likely to identify as transgender women. Reisner and colleagues showed that 19% of transgender women in their cohort had been incarcerated at some point.[16] Further, this cohort was more likely to be people of color, have lower income, lower education status, receive public insurance, or not have insurance compared with those without a history of incarceration. In this study, Black transgender women were at 3 times greater risk of incarceration than White transgender women. Other social vulnerabilities resulting in increased reports of incarceration are given in **Table 1**.

The US survey of federal and state prison inmates in 2016 indicated that 0.3% of inmates self-identified as transgender or identified with a gender different from their sex assigned at birth.[17] Although a small representation of the survey, the individuals who identified as transgender were more likely to be people of color and younger than the general inmate population.[17,18] A news report from NBC News in 2020 found 4,890 transgender prisoners living in state prisons across the United States[19] This is similar to previous estimates of individuals with gender dysphoria in US male prisons at 3000 to 4000.[20]

Transgender women were more likely to report longer lengths of incarceration than transgender men or gender-nonconforming individuals.[2] Of those who reported incarceration, Black and American Indian respondents, those with lower household income and less educational attainment were more likely to report longer lengths of incarceration.

For their health care, these individuals are likely to be seen by internal corrections facility providers but may also be seen by endocrinologists through a partnership between an academic institution and a corrections facility or outsourced to private providers.[21] Specialty care, such as endocrinology, often requires transportation to an academic health care institution for treatment or a designated telehealth clinic. Understanding the structural challenges to gender-affirming care in the corrections environment will allow the endocrinologist to navigate the complex correctional health care system. The barriers to gender-affirming care and surgery will be highlighted below.

After Incarceration

According to the Federal Bureau of Prisons, > 39,000 inmates were released in 2022.[22] Approximately, 16% of transgender people (21% of transgender women and 10% of transgender men) in a large national survey reported a past history of incarceration, but this may be > 50% in some cohorts (ie, cohorts that focus on transgender women).[2,23] These individuals will present to the clinic with many having been denied health care (12%) or hormone affirming care (17%), prevented from continuing hormone therapy during incarceration (37%), and having been the victims of physical (16%) or sexual assault (15%) from other inmates or corrections officers whereas in jail or prison.[1,2] Health care denial whereas incarcerated (25%) in a cohort of transfeminine spectrum individuals was associated with age, public health insurance, gender-affirming hormone use, substance use as a coping mechanism, and identifying as Asian/Pacific Islander versus non-Hispanic White or women.[16] This same cohort reported a number of health vulnerabilities, including smoking, HIV-positive status, substance abuse to cope, assault, and sex work, compared with those without a history of jail/prison. From 2017 to 2020, the rate of victimization against transgender people was 2.5x that of nontransgender people who are incarcerated.[24] A history of incarceration in a population of young transgender women in 2 large urban cities was significantly associated with low self-esteem, polysubstance use, victimization, and intimate partner violence.[23] Transgender people who reported gender-based abuse during incarceration were more likely to report attempting suicide in their lifetime.[25] Prior jail/prison was associated with fewer social (ie, health or financial) support networks after release and utilization of health care services (ie, emergency department, urgent care) at higher rates than nontransgender individuals.[26,27] Perhaps most importantly, the medical history should include a question about any history of incarceration. Addressing these concerns is outside the scope of this article, but there are opportunities to be prepared to provide a trauma-informed approach to care, ensure the individual is connected to primary preventative care, and allocate resources such as mental health care, case management, and social work.[9,28] These individuals may disconnect from care because of negative prior experiences with health care that violated trust.[1]

DISCUSSION

Standards of Care (SOC) for the health and psychological well-being of transgender individuals have been published by the World Professional Association for Transgender Health (WPATH).[29] Currently in version 8 (SOC-8), it provides specific recommendations for transgender care in institutional environments. It states that all recommendations made in the SOC-8 be applied equally to people living in institutions. Specifically for institutions such as correction facilities, the SOC-8 recommends that staff receive training in gender diversity, always use chosen names and pronouns, and provide appropriate clothing/grooming items and a private shower/toilet if requested. With regards to housing, the SOC-8 encourages an individual's housing preference, gender identity, gender expression, and safety to be considered for housing and not just the sex assigned at birth. The housing of transgender individuals should be safe without segregating or isolating individuals. For medical professionals specifically, it is recommended that they provide gender affirming hormone therapy and surgical treatments without delay.

Correction facilities' ability to meet these SOC is complicated. The legal system and correction facility policies vary in their support of gender-affirming care. The care that a transgender person may or may not receive may be wholly dependent upon the state in which they are incarcerated. Although the corrections system can pose harm to transgender inmates, which will be discussed, it may be the first opportunity to access health care by this marginalized community.

One of the challenges regarding gender-affirming care is legal precedent. Most courts and Congress have taken a binary definition of gender. The Seventh, Eighth, and Tenth Circuit Courts of Appeal have ruled in favor of binary definitions concerning sexual discrimination brought under Title VII of the Civil Rights Act of 1964.[30,31] The American with Disabilities Act and the Federal Rehabilitation Act exclude transgender from the protections they offer. The Ninth Circuit Court of Appeals has ruled in favor of expanding legal protections for transgender individuals by adding gender identity to the concept of sex.[32,33]

Inconsistent policies across corrections are a barrier to caring for transgender inmates. A 2017 review of US Department of Corrections (DOC) policies looked at access to counseling services, hormone initiation, hormone continuation, and gender-affirming surgery.[32] Thirty-seven states allow for a counseling appointment to assist with coping with gender dysphoria or exploring gender identity. This is considered "adequate care" and where most DOC care regarding gender identity stops. Seven states do not allow counseling and 6 states have unknown policies. Only 13 states allow hormone initiation while incarcerated. Twenty-one states allow the continuation of hormone therapy upon incarceration, whereas 20 states do not allow the continuation of hormone therapy. In 10 states, the use of hormone therapy is unknown. Only 7 states allow gender-affirming surgery.

Barriers to Gender-Affirming Care

Gender-affirming care faces several barriers that are structural, interpersonal, and educational. Structural barriers are primarily policies that, while potentially well-meaning with their focus on physical safety and security, result in further victimization of transgender inmates. Interpersonal barriers include corrections and medical staff personal bias regarding transgender care. The greatest individual barrier is a lack of cultural and clinical competence.

Prison culture is a structural barrier to gender-affirming care. Prison assignments are based on binary definitions of gender and inmates are housed according to the sex assigned at birth or genital status. Upon incarceration, some individuals undergo strip searches to identify their genital status. This can be a dysphoric and stressful experience for a transgender person.[34] Transgender women inmates may be further victimized by the hierarchical structure of prison, which is based on hypermasculine culture.[35] Transgender inmates with feminized characteristics are more likely to be physically and sexually assaulted.[36] For safety, transgender inmates may seek placement, or be involuntarily placed, in segregation units. In addition to the social isolation and loss of liberties in these units, policies exist requiring frequent or mandatory strip searches or pat downs to leave the segregation units to visit the medical wing. Some inmates may choose to forgo medical visits to avoid this.[37,38] Lastly, in a survey of > 1,200 LGBTQ prisoners, 15% of 950 inmates self-identified as transgender women (no report on % transgender men). Seventy-eight percent of transgender, nonbinary, and Two-Spirit respondents reported hiding their gender identity while incarcerated, resulting in emotional distress.[39]

Because initiation of hormone affirming care is not allowed in 37/50 states, transgender inmates may need a previous diagnosis to receive treatment and previous prescription evidence of hormone therapy to continue it while incarcerated.[32,40,41] Transgender inmates indicated that less than half had a prior diagnosis of gender dysphoria or gender identity disorder and a third were denied seeking this diagnosis while incarcerated.[39] Because transgender individuals are often marginalized, many obtain unconventional medical care, including sourcing hormones without a prescription (often termed street hormones), further limiting their ability to continue care while incarcerated.[39,42] Frequent prison transfers can lead to a lack of continuity of care.[43] These situations can result in the abrupt cessation of hormone therapy upon incarceration.[44] The challenges of hormone disruption, including hot flashes, facial hair, resumption of erections, or menses, can be distressing to inmates. Budgetary concerns are also a barrier, with medical providers identifying the cost of hormone therapy as prohibitive.[41] With a limited budget, the controversial nature of hormone therapy results in other health care priorities taking precedence.

An interpersonal barrier to care is custodial and medical staff bias toward transgender inmates. A 2009 survey of transgender and gender nonconforming inmates in Pennsylvania reported that 42% thought that their medical needs were not taken seriously by medical staff.[45] In a large LGBT inmate survey, only 21% of transgender inmates indicated that they were allowed access to undergarments and cosmetic needs that aligned with their gender identity.[39] In a survey of 20 correctional health providers, providers identified that correctional staff had a bias against transgender inmates and the health providers. This impacted their ability to provide medical care.[41] Providers thought they had to balance advocacy for the inmates with the views of custodial staff, who often viewed transgender medical care as unnecessary. An adversarial relationship between custodial staff and medical providers may result in inmates not being brought to appointments or having group sessions canceled.[41]

Lack of cultural and clinical competence in transgender care is an educational barrier to care. Correctional staff often have little training in transgender competent care.[43] This is not vastly different from clinical providers, including those outside of corrections. In a national survey, up to 50% of transgender individuals thought the need to educate their providers about their care.[1] The authors of this article have published a survey of internal medicine residents at an academic medical center and established primary providers who worked in corrections on their prior transgender learning experience and patient exposure. Although 88% of established providers reported medically caring for at least 1 transgender patient, 61% stated they had no exposure to transgender teaching.[46] One study noted that clinical corrections staff thought they had to independently seek out training outside of the corrections.[41] At the same time, providers think unprepared to provide gender affirming care. One physician noted, "I have a few [transgender] patients. I never know if you're supposed to titrate [hormones]...how you approach dosing. I usually just keep them what they are on."[41] The same study that surveyed clinical staff in corrections noted a lack of cultural competency by medical staff, who would not use appropriate pronouns or preferred names. A recurring theme from some clinical providers was that transgender inmates were "flag-waving or showing off in a sex-segregated system" and being manipulative to gain special treatment.

Barriers to Gender-Affirming Surgery

Gender-affirming surgery has only been offered to inmates in response to litigation. Procedures include orchiectomy, penectomy, and vaginoplasty. Gender-affirming surgery can be highly effective in treating anatomic gender dysphoria, or the intense distress about the incongruence between external genitals and gender identity.[20]

The WPATH SOC-8 explicitly states that all provisions in the SOC-8 be applied equally to all people living in institutions, including incarceration.[29] There are 7 standard eligibility requirements outlined for gender-affirming surgery in the WPATH SOC-8. As discussed previously, incarcerated transgender people may have difficulty accessing gender counseling, may not have providers with experience or education to counsel through informed consent and effects on reproduction, and may not have access to fertility preservation resources, which are costly. Lastly, policy and structural challenges may result in barriers to initiating or continuing hormone affirming care to provide stability in hormone exposure such that surgical results can be individualized and maximized for the individual. Although ethical agreement with this principle is easy, the lived reality that incarcerated transgender individuals face is more complex.

Forty percent of transgender inmates in a large LGBTQ inmate survey indicated that they were denied access to requested gender-affirming surgeries.[39] One case series noted 4 inmates who identified as transgender women and attempted or completed surgical self-treatment (SST) (autocastration with or without autopenectomy) for severe gender dysphoria.[47] All had requested gendering affirming hormone therapy but were denied. In a setting of lost hope, the individuals proceeded with SST with the explicit goal of reducing testosterone levels and reducing their anatomic gender dysphoria. All 4 inmates declined testosterone supplementation that was subsequently offered to them by the DOC. The author notes that in prisons where gender affirming hormone therapy is available, SST has not been reported.

Role of the Endocrinologist

The participation of the endocrinologist in the care of an incarcerated transgender person likely depends on the state that they practice in, their participation in the care of incarcerated individuals and correction facility access to endocrinologic care. Endocrinologists, particularly those within academic teaching institutions, may consider establishing and participating in correction clinics.[21] Collaboration between a corrections facility and an academic institution aligns with the academic mission to serve marginalized populations. These are excellent training opportunities for medical students, residents, and fellows and are chances to address complex care, population health, and health care delivery. The endocrinologist can augment the knowledge/experience gaps of corrections staff regarding informed consent, readiness for gender-affirming care, initiation or continuation of gender-affirming care, and aid in identifying care gaps.

Endocrinologists can also participate in advancing research, education, and training. The United Nations Development Program challenges that “without systematic data collection and monitoring it is impossible to identify and address current gaps, and to ensure trans[gender] prisoners’ rights to dignity, health and life.”[48] The 2015 US Trans Survey is being updated. A new survey (open from October 19, 2022 to December 5, 2022) included updated information on interactions with police and prisons that will be valuable to reassess the scope of the situation as well as significant changes in reported experiences.[49]

Establishing relationships with corrections institutions to assist in transgender competent care training may be possible. White Hughto and colleagues piloted 4 learning modules that were successful in providing transgender competent education to corrections staff, and those staff reported that they would recommend the training to others.[50] Staff training can impact the quality of care. In a study of 12 New York City jails following a survey of incarcerated transgender individuals, a quality improvement initiative incorporated LGBT training and a new transgender care policy for all medical, nursing, and mental health staff. After 3 months, patient complaints dropped by 50%. After 6 months, complaints dropped to zero.[51] In another study in New England, a training intervention improved transgender competent care for correctional health care providers and their willingness to provide gender-affirming care to incarcerated transgender people.[52]

SUMMARY

As transgender health care becomes increasingly politicized, and states enact barriers to safe legal health care for transgender individuals, a marginalized community faces further victimization.[53,54] Discrimination in social determinants of health and increased rates of incarceration compared with the general population, combined with inconsistent correctional policies, pose challenges to the incarcerated individual who seeks gender affirming care. By educating endocrinologists on the structural, interpersonal, and educational barriers to care, we hope to empower providers to navigate these complexities to improve the health of transgender individuals.

CLINICS CARE POINTS

- Transgender people are at higher risk for justice system involvement.
- The WPATH Standards of Care-8 state that all institutionalized transgender individuals receive gender affirming care.
- Inconsistent legal policies and systemic barriers in the US Correctional System result in variable gender affirming care.
- Endocrinologists educated on the structural, interpersonal, and educational barriers to care can be empowered to navigate these complexities to improve the health of incarcerated transgender individuals.

DISCLOSURE

R. Malek and E. Lamos have no commercial or financial disclosures. Support for this manuscript comes in part from a “Building Trust through Diversity, Health Care Equity, Inclusion and Diagnostic Excellence in Internal Medicine Training” grant sponsored by the Alliance for Academic Internal Medicine (AAIM), the American Board of Medicine (ABIM), the ABIM Foundation, the American College of Physicians (ACP), and the Josiah Macy Jr. Foundation. M. Sarmiento is an employee of YesCare Corporation.

REFERENCES

1. James SE, Herman JL, Rankin S, et al. The report of the 2015. U.S. Transgender Survey.; 2016. https://transequality.org/sites/default/files/docs/usts/USTS-Full-Report-Dec17.pdf.
2. Grant JMLTJHJHJKM. Injustice at Every Turn. A Report of the National Transgender Discrimination Survey.; 2011. Available at: https://transequality.org/sites/default/files/docs/resources/NTDS_Report.pdf.
3. Reisner SL, Poteat T, Keatley J, et al. Global health burden and needs of transgender populations: a review. Lancet 2016;388(10042):412–36.

4. White Hughto JM, Reisner SL, Pachankis JE. Transgender stigma and health: A critical review of stigma determinants, mechanisms, and interventions. Soc Sci Med 2015;147:222–31.
5. CDC. HIV and Transgender People. Published 2022. Accessed February 10, 2022. https://www.cdc.gov/hiv/group/gender/transgender/index.html.
6. Peitzmeier SM, Khullar K, Reisner SL, et al. Pap test use is lower among female-to-male patients than non-transgender women. Am J Prev Med 2014;47(6): 808–12.
7. Oladeru OT, Ma SJ, Miccio JA, et al. Breast and Cervical Cancer Screening Disparities in Transgender People. Am J Clin Oncol 2022;45(3):116–21.
8. van Hout MC, Kewley S, Hillis A. Contemporary transgender health experience and health situation in prisons: A scoping review of extant published literature (2000-2019). Int J Transgend Health 2020;21(3):258–306.
9. Hughto JMW, Reisner SL, Kershaw TS, et al. A multisite, longitudinal study of risk factors for incarceration and impact on mental health and substance use among young transgender women in the USA. J Public Health 2019;41(1):100–9.
10. Hughto JMW, Clark KA, Daken K, et al. Victimization Within and Beyond the Prison Walls: A Latent Profile Analysis of Transgender and Gender Diverse Adults. J Interpers Violence 2022;37(23–24):NP23075–106.
11. Deal C, Doshi RD, Gonzales G. Gender Minority Youth Experiencing Homelessness and Corresponding Health Disparities. J Adolesc Health 2023. https://doi.org/10.1016/j.jadohealth.2022.11.229.
12. Nadal KL, Davidoff KC, Fujii-Doe W. Transgender women and the sex work industry: roots in systemic, institutional, and interpersonal discrimination. J Trauma & Dissociation 2014;15(2):169–83.
13. Harvey TD, Hughto JMW, Clark KA. Availability of Accessible Representative Health Data to Examine Sexual and Gender Minority Disparities in Incarceration and Its Health Implications in the United States, 2010-2020. LGBT Health 2022; 9(2):81–93.
14. Beck A. PREA Data Collection Activities, 2015.; 2015. Available at: https://bjs.ojp.gov/content/pub/pdf/pdca15.pdf.
15. Cotter R. Length of Incarderation and Recidivism.; 2022. Available at: https://www.ussc.gov/sites/default/files/pdf/research-and-publications/research-publications/2022/20220621_Recidivsm-SentLength.pdf.
16. Reisner SL, Bailey Z, Sevelius J. Racial/ethnic disparities in history of incarceration, experiences of victimization, and associated health indicators among transgender women in the U.S. Women Health 2014;54(8):750–67.
17. Beatty, LG; Snell T. Profle of Prison Inmates, 2016.; 2021. Available at: https://bjs.ojp.gov/content/pub/pdf/ppi16.pdf.
18. Herring, T; Widra E. What the Survey of Prison Inmates tells us about trans people in state prison. Prison Policy Initiative. Published 2022 Available at: https://www.prisonpolicy.org/blog/2022/03/31/transgender_incarceration/. Accessed February 10, 2023.
19. Sosin K. Few transgender prisoners are housed according to their identity — putting many in danger. NBC News; 2020. https://www.nbcnews.com/feature/nbc-out/transgender-women-are-nearly-always-incarcerated-men-s-putting-many-n1142436.
20. Osborne CS, Lawrence AA. Male Prison Inmates With Gender Dysphoria: When Is Sex Reassignment Surgery Appropriate? Arch Sex Behav 2016;45(7):1649–63.
21. Trestman RL, Ferguson W, Dickert J. Behind bars: the compelling case for academic health centers partnering with correctional facilities. Acad Med 2015;90(1):16–9.

22. Federal Beueau of Prisons. Release Numbers. Published 2023. Accessed February 10, 2023. Available at: https://www.bop.gov/about/statistics/statistics_inmate_releases.jsp.
23. Brennan J, Kuhns LM, Johnson AK, et al. Syndemic theory and HIV-related risk among young transgender women: the role of multiple, co-occurring health problems and social marginalization. Am J Public Health 2012;102(9):1751–7.
24. Truman JL, Ph D, Morgan RE, Ph D, Statisticians BJS. Violent Victimization by Sexual Orientation and Gender Identity, 2017–2020. 2022;(June):1-22. Available at: https://bjs.ojp.gov/content/pub/pdf/vvsogi1720.pdf.
25. Drakeford L. Correctional Policy and Attempted Suicide Among Transgender Individuals. J Correct Health Care 2018;24(2):171–82.
26. Scheidell JD, Kapadia F, Turpin RE, et al. Incarceration, Social Support Networks, and Health among Black Sexual Minority Men and Transgender Women: Evidence from the HPTN 061 Study. Int J Environ Res Public Health 2022;19(19). https://doi.org/10.3390/ijerph191912064.
27. Walsh KB, Will J, Chyten-Brennan J. Community Health Care Utilization Patterns in Transgender Individuals Who Have Been Incarcerated. J Correct Health Care 2023. https://doi.org/10.1089/jchc.21.10.0120.
28. Sevelius JM, Castro DA, Warri V, et al. Adapting and Implementing an Evidence-Based Reentry Intervention for Incarcerated Transgender Women: Lessons Learned. J Correct Health Care 2023. https://doi.org/10.1089/jchc.21.12.0132.
29. Coleman E, Radix AE, Bouman WP, et al. Standards of Care for the Health of Transgender and Gender Diverse People, Version 8. Int J Transgend Health 2022;23(Suppl 1):S1–259.
30. Lloyd A. Defining the Human: Are Transgender People Strangers to the Law? Berk J Gend Law Justice 2005;20(1):150–95.
31. Twing SD, Williams T. Title VII's Transgender Trajectory: An Analysis of Whether Transgender People Are a Protected Class under the Term "Sex" and Practical Implications of Inclusion. Texas Journal on Civil Liberties & Civil Rights 2010; 15:173–203. Available at: https://sites.utexas.edu/tjclcr/files/2022/11/Twing-Williams_Title-VIIs-Transgender-Trajectory.pdf.
32. Routh D, Abess G, Makin D, et al. Transgender Inmates in Prisons. Int J Offender Ther Comp Criminol 2017;61(6):645–66.
33. Colopy TW. Setting gender identity free: expanding treatment for transsexual inmates. Health Matrix Clevel 2012;22(1):227–72.
34. Wesp L. Transgender patients and the physical examination. In: Deutsch M, editor. Guidelines for the primary and gender-affirming care of transgender and gender Nonbinary people. 2nd edition; 2016. Available at: https://transcare.ucsf.edu/guidelines/physical-examination. Accessed February 12, 2023.
35. Lutze FE, Murphy DW. Ultramasculine prison environments and inmates' adjustment: It's time to move beyond the "boys will be boys" paradigm. Justice Q JQ 1999;16(4):709–33.
36. Mazza, GJ; Wilkinson, RA; Christensen GSA. Report on Sexual Victimization in Prisons and Jails.; 2012. Available at: http://www.ojp.usdoj.gov/reviewpanel/reviewpanel.htm.
37. Smith W, Smith WE. (2012). In the Footsteps of Johnson V. California: Why Classification and Segregation of Transgender Inmates Warrants Heightened Scrutiny. J Gend Race Justice 2012;15:689. Available at: https://heinonline.org/HOL/LandingPage?handle=hein.journals/jgrj15&div=29&id=&page=.

38. S S. "One is Not Born, But Becomes a Woman": A Fourteenth Amendment Argument in Support of Housing Male-to-Female Transgender Inmates in Female Facilities. 15 U Pa J Const L. Published online 2013:1259.
39. Lydon J, Carrington K, Low H, et al. Coming out of Concrete Closets: a report on Black & Pink's national LGBTQ prisoner survey. Black and Pink; 2015. Available at: http://arks.princeton.edu/ark:/88435/dsp018p58pg71d.
40. von Dresner KS, Underwood LA, Suarez E, et al. Providing counseling for transgendered inmates: A survey of correctional services. Int J Behav Consult Ther (IJBCT) 2013;7:38–44.
41. Clark KA, White Hughto JM, Pachankis JE. "What's the right thing to do?" Correctional healthcare providers' knowledge, attitudes and experiences caring for transgender inmates. Soc Sci Med 2017;193:80–9.
42. Stroumsa D, Crissman HP, Dalton VK, et al. Insurance Coverage and Use of Hormones Among Transgender Respondents to a National Survey. Ann Fam Med 2020;18(6):528–34.
43. Tarzwell S, Tarzwell S. The gender liens are marked with razor wire: Addressing state prison policies and practices for the management of transgender prisoners. Colum Hum Rts 2006;38:167. Available at: https://heinonline.org/HOL/LandingPage?handle=hein.journals/colhr38&div=9&id=&page=.
44. McCauley E, Eckstrand K, Desta B, et al. Exploring Healthcare Experiences for Incarcerated Individuals Who Identify as Transgender in a Southern Jail. Transgend Health 2018;3(1):34–41.
45. Emmer, P; Lowe, A; Marshall R. This Is a Prison, Glitter Is Not Allowed: Experiences of Trans and Gender Variant People in Pennsylvania's Prison Systems.; 2011. https://heartsonawire.org/wp-content/uploads/2018/09/thisisaprison.pdf.
46. Malek R, Sarmiento M, Lamos E. ODP410 Exposure to Transgender Teaching in Internal Medicine Residents and Established Providers. J Endocr Soc 2022; 6(Supplement_1):A660–1.
47. Brown GR. Autocastration and Autopenectomy as Surgical Self-Treatment in Incarcerated Persons with Gender Identity Disorder. Int J Transgenderism 2010;12(1):31–9.
48. Transgender Health and Human Rights.; 2013. Available at: https://www.undp.org/sites/g/files/zskgke326/files/publications/Trans Health & Human Rights.pdf.
49. U.S. Trans Survey 2022. Available at: https://www.ustranssurvey.org/Accessed February 10, 2023.
50. White Hughto JM, Clark KA. Designing a Transgender Health Training for Correctional Health Care Providers: A Feasibility Study. Prison J 2019;99(3):329–42.
51. Jaffer M, Ayad J, Tungol JG, et al. Improving Transgender Healthcare in the New York City Correctional System. LGBT Health 2016;3(2):116–21.
52. White Hughto JM, Clark KA, Altice FL, et al. Improving correctional healthcare providers' ability to care for transgender patients: Development and evaluation of a theory-driven cultural and clinical competence intervention. Soc Sci Med 2017;195:159–69.
53. Hughes LD, Kidd KM, Gamarel KE, et al. "These Laws Will Be Devastating": Provider Perspectives on Legislation Banning Gender-Affirming Care for Transgender Adolescents. J Adolesc Health 2021;69(6):976–82.
54. West S. Targeted by Politicians, trans youth struggle with growing fear and mental health concerns. Kaiser Health News; 2022. Available at: https://khn.org/news/article/transgender-youth-mental-health-targeted-by-politicians/. Accessed February 14, 2023.

Disparities in Access to High-Volume Surgeons and Specialized Care

Terry P. Gao, MD, Rebecca L. Green, MD, Lindsay E. Kuo, MD, MBA*

KEYWORDS

• Volume • Outcome • Disparity in access • Quality • Endocrine surgery
• High-volume surgeons • High-volume centers • Specialized care

KEY POINTS

- A significant volume–outcome relationship exists within endocrine surgery.
- The volume–outcome relationship is multifactorial: high-volume (HV) centers may have specialized/multidisciplinary care coordination and increased experience in managing specific diseases, and high-volume surgeons gain clinical and technical proficiency over time, resulting in superior outcomes.
- Significant gaps in utilization of HV care exist. Systems and patient factors may contribute to decreased HV access for some populations, leading to decreased utilization and poorer surgical outcomes.

INTRODUCTION

Perioperative and surgical management of diseases involving the thyroid, parathyroid, adrenal glands, and pancreatic neuroendocrine tumors has become increasingly complex, involving multimodal imaging, minimally invasive techniques, and intraoperative hormone or radio-guided monitoring.[1] Despite the field's growing complexity, a majority of endocrine surgeries are still performed by surgeons without specific expertise.[2] Since Birkmeyer and colleagues[3,4] first established a relationship between increased center and surgeon volume and decreased mortality for cardiovascular and cancer operations, numerous studies have asserted the positive correlation between higher volumes (HV) and improved patient outcomes.[5–8] This relationship holds true for thyroidectomy, parathyroidectomy, adrenalectomy, and pancreatectomy, and spans functional, nonfunctional, benign, and malignant disease.[9–11] However, significant gaps in access to HV care exist. In the following sections, we discuss current definitions for HV centers and surgeons with respect to thyroid, parathyroid, adrenal, and

Department of General Surgery, Temple University Hospital, 3401 North Broad Street, Zone C, 4th Floor, Philadelphia, PA 19140, USA
* Corresponding author.
E-mail address: Lindsay.Kuo@tuhs.temple.edu

Endocrinol Metab Clin N Am 52 (2023) 689–703
https://doi.org/10.1016/j.ecl.2023.05.006

pancreatic neuroendocrine surgeries, and examine the impact of the associated disparities on access to HV care.

HIGH-VOLUME SURGEON AND CENTER DEFINITIONS AND ASSOCIATED OUTCOMES

The current definitions for HV surgical care for thyroid, parathyroid, adrenal, and pancreatic neuroendocrine disease are highly variable. Additionally, the published literature on this subject is often nonspecific to surgical indication. For parathyroid surgery, most of the literature on volume or on disparities in access focuses on primary hyperparathyroidism or parathyroid disease in general, with little distinction between specific parathyroid pathologies. For adrenal surgery, the literature addresses benign or malignant adrenal disease, with a paucity of data addressing specific functional adrenal tumors (ie, Cushing's or primary aldosteronism). For pancreatic surgery, most of the literature focuses on pancreatic adenocarcinoma or makes little distinction between the types of pancreatic neoplasms encountered. Consequently, the volume definitions for these sections will discuss gland-specific surgery as a whole.

Thyroid Surgery

The current thresholds for a HV thyroid surgeon range from $\geq$23 to $\geq$100 thyroidectomies per year.[6,12] Inconsistency in this definition makes it difficult to compare results between studies and analyze the true impact of a HV surgeon on patient outcomes.[13] Recent meta-analyses have identified greater than 100 thyroidectomies annually for a single center as a threshold for a HV center.[5,14] Notably, an individual surgeon's experience rather than a center's experience[6,13,14] has been found to correlate more significantly with complications. There is no association between surgical specialty (endocrine surgeon, head and neck surgeon, or other) and surgical outcomes.[15–18]

Increased surgical volumes are associated with superior thyroidectomy-specific outcomes for all surgical thyroid disease. HV surgeons have lower rates of recurrent laryngeal nerve (RLN) injury,[5,6,12] lower rates of clinically significant postoperative hypocalcemia,[5,6] and reduced postoperative length of stay (LOS).[5,19] Graves' disease—an independent risk factor for postoperative complications—is associated with higher incidences of RLN injury and hypocalcemia when thyroidectomy is performed by a low volume (LV) surgeon.[12,20] Patients with Graves' disease who received surgery at HV centers experienced lower rates of postoperative hematoma (1.4% vs. 3.1%), hypocalcemia (7.0% vs. 13.9%), tracheostomy (0.2% vs. 1.3%), and major medical complications (1.2% vs. 3.4%; $P < 0.01$ for all).[20]

For thyroid cancer surgery, both high surgeon and center volumes are associated with improved cancer-specific outcomes. Thyroid cancer surgery by HV surgeons is associated with lower rates of cancer recurrence, whereas surgery performed by LV surgeons is an independent prognostic factor for shorter local recurrence-free survival.[21] Notably, no significant differences in long-term oncologic outcomes (ie, distant metastasis-free survival or cancer-specific mortality-free survival) were observed between HV and LV surgeons.[21] Thyroid cancer surgery at HV centers is associated with lower odds of postoperative hematoma, hypocalcemia, vocal-cord paralysis, tracheostomy, and major medical complications compared to LV centers.[20]

As more thyroidectomies in the United States are performed in the outpatient setting, utilization of inpatient data alone may confound reported results with selection bias, as patients undergoing inpatient procedures may have more severe or complex disease.[22] In one of the few studies on outpatient thyroidectomies, the majority were performed at HV centers (61% vs. 27%) by HV surgeons (48% vs. 24%).[23] Of note, HV surgeons were independently predictive of same-day discharge and a decreased likelihood of rehospitalization,[23] whereas postoperative complications were significantly higher in outpatients managed by LV surgeons.[24]

Given the abundance of data associating improved postoperative outcomes with increased surgical volume, the American Association of Endocrine Surgeons (AAES) recommends that, when possible, thyroidectomy should be performed by a HV thyroid surgeon,[25] and some authors recommend that thyroidectomy in complex patients (ie, Graves' or cancer) be performed solely at HV centers to mitigate the increased risk of complications.[12] The relationship between center and surgeon volume and associated outcomes is shown in **Table 1**.

Parathyroid Surgery

The definition of a HV parathyroid surgeon ranges from a minimum of 20 to 100 parathyroidectomies a year.[26–28] Surgeons who perform less than 2 to 20 parathyroidectomies a year have been considered LV in the literature,[27,29] whereas the AAES and European Society of Endocrine Surgeons define a LV surgeon as performing less than 10 to 15 parathyroidectomies a year.[26,30]

Superior outcomes are evident after parathyroidectomy by HV parathyroid surgeons compared to LV surgeons.[8,11] Higher rates of complications,[27–29,31,32] reoperation for persistent disease,[32] persistent hypercalcemia,[33] longer postoperative LOS,[27,28,32] and higher costs[27,28] are seen after parathyroidectomy by LV compared to HV surgeons. Though surgeon volume appears to have a greater impact on outcomes after parathyroidectomy than center volume,[34,35] center volume also impacts outcomes after parathyroidectomy, with higher rates of cure in HV centers,[36,37] and higher rates of reoperation and persistent hyperparathyroidism in LV centers.[36–39] This was further explored in a single-center study that looked at referral patterns for reoperative parathyroidectomy: 95% of patients referred from LV centers had an avoidable reoperation for persistent primary hyperparathyroidism (ie, missed gland in normal anatomic location) compared to 41% of patients referred from HV centers.[40] The relationship between center and surgeon volume and associated outcomes is shown in **Table 2**.

Adrenal Surgery

For both benign and malignant adrenal disease, surgeons who perform greater than 4 to 7 adrenalectomies per year have been considered HV.[9,41–46] For benign disease, the definition of HV centers ranges from greater than 14 to greater than 65 adrenalectomies per year.[9,42,43,47] For adrenal cortical carcinoma (ACC), the definition of a HV center is poorly defined, ranging from greater than 4 to greater than 10 ACC cases per year.[48–50] This small volume of cases required for HV designation is likely due to the rarity of ACC.[51] Unfortunately, less than 50% of ACC are managed at HV centers,[49,50,52] most of which are academic cancer centers (91%–94%).

For both benign and malignant adrenal disease, increased surgical volumes are associated with improved outcomes. Surgical management of benign adrenal disease by HV adrenal surgeons is not only associated with lower rates of postoperative complications (10.2%–11.6% vs. 16.4%–18.8%),[42–44] but also lower rates of perioperative mortality (0.6% vs. 1.3–2.4%)[44,45] and shorter hospital LOS (2.7–3.9 vs. 4.2–6.0 days)[42,43,45] in comparison to LV surgeons. Improved outcomes for HV adrenal surgeons are seen regardless of surgeon specialty (urologist, endocrine surgeon, or other specialized general surgeon).[44] Adrenalectomy at HV centers is similarly associated with lower rates of complications (6.7%–22.2% vs. 16.8%–36.6%)[9,42,43] and shorter LOS (4.1 vs. 5.3 days).[43] The relationship between surgeon volume and associated outcomes after adrenalectomy for benign disease is shown in **Table 3**.

Table 1
The impact of surgeon and center volume on outcomes after thyroidectomy

Author, Year	Annual Volume Thresholds	Significant Outcomes
Surgeon volume		
Sosa et al,[88] 1998	• A: 1–9 • B: 10–29 • C: 30–100 • D: ≥100	• Mean LOS was shortest for HV surgeons (1.4 vs. 1.7 vs. 1.7 vs. 1.9 days) • Complication rates were lowest for HV surgeons (5.1% vs. 6.1% vs. 6.1% vs. 8.6%)
Gourin et al,[5] 2010	• Low: ≤ 3 • Intermediate: 4–24 • High: ≥ 24	• Complications were less likely for HV surgeons (RLN injury: OR 0.46, 95% CI 0.32–0.69, hypocalcemia: OR 0.49, 95% CI 0.41–0.57) • Prolonged LOS was less likely for HV surgeons (OR 0.44, 95% CI 0.41–0.47)
Loyo,[6] 2013	• Very Low: ≤ 3 • Low: 4–9 • Intermediate: 9–23 • High: >23	• Postoperative complications were less likely for HV surgeons (OR 0.73, 95% CI 0.63–0.86) • Nonhome discharge was less likely for HV than LV surgeons (OR 0.35, 95% CI 0.25–0.51)
Kandil et al,[12] 2013	• Low: ≤ 10 • Intermediate: 10–99 • High: ≥ 100	• Surgery for Graves' disease was independently associated with postoperative complications compared to surgery for benign disease when performed by LV (OR 1.39, 95% CI 1.08–1.79) but not for HV surgeons (OR 1.07, 95% CI 0.62–1.83)
Hauch et al,[65] 2014	• Low: ≤ 10 • High: >99	• Postoperative complications after total thyroidectomy were more likely for LV surgeons (OR 1.53, 95% CI 1.12–2.11)
Liang et al,[19] 2016	• Low: 1–70 • High: >70	• Mean LOS was shorter for HV surgeons (0.2 days [6.3%] shorter) • Mean costs were lower for HV surgeons ($17.6 [1.6%] lower)
Kim et al,[21] 2018	• Low: <100 • High: ≥ 100	• Likelihood of structural recurrence after thyroidectomy for papillary thyroid cancer was greater for LV surgeons (OR 1.46, 95% CI 1.08–1.96) • No difference in distant metastasis and disease specific mortality seen between surgeon volume (*P* = 0.242 and 0.288)
Center Volume		
Gourin et al, 2010	• Low: ≤ 22 • Intermediate: 23–100 • High: ≥ 100	• Center volume was not significantly associated with risk of postoperative complications after adjusting for surgeon volume
Loyo[6] 2013	• Very low: ≤ 25 • Low: 26–42 • Intermediate: 43–76 • High: >76	• Center volume was not significantly associated with risk of postoperative complications after adjusting for surgeon volume

(*continued on next page*)

Table 1
(*continued*)

Author, Year	Annual Volume Thresholds	Significant Outcomes
Liang et al,[19] 2016	• Low: 1–200 • High: >200	• Mean LOS was shorter for HV centers (0.2 days [6.3%] shorter) • Mean costs were lower for HV centers ($39.6 [3.6%] lower)

Abbreviations: HR, hazard ratio; HV, high volume; LOS, length of stay; LV, low volume; OR, odds ratio.

In the management of ACC, HV centers are more likely than LV centers to operate on ACC when resectable, whereas LV centers are more likely to offer nonoperative management; HV centers are also more likely to perform a radical resection.[53,54] Accordingly, surgery at HV centers is associated with 33% lower odds of positive margins.[50] This is vital, as complete surgical resection offers the only potential for cure.[25] Receipt of chemotherapy including mitotane is more common at HV centers compared to LV centers (35%–44% vs. 24%–31%).[52,53] This optimized treatment approach—surgery resulting in a microscopically negative resection margin (R0), followed by chemotherapy—may be related to the presence of multidisciplinary care teams at HV centers,[25,55] and may explain the lower rates of local recurrence (6% vs. 19%) and longer recurrence-free survival (mean 25 vs. 10 months) at HV versus LV centers.[48] However, despite the more aggressive treatment approach at HV centers, no differences in overall survival have been reported for patients treated at LV versus HV centers, likely related to the aggressive nature of ACC.[49,56]

Pancreatic Surgery

The paucity of data addressing HV surgical care specifically for pancreatic neuroendocrine tumors necessitates volume definitions herein to pancreatic surgery as a whole. An HV center performs greater than 50 to greater than 100 pancreatic surgeries annually[57,58] and an HV surgeon performs greater than 5 to greater than 20 annually.[3,4] Notably, most pancreatic surgeries occur at LV centers.[59]

Pancreatic surgeries performed at HV centers are associated with reduced overall morbidity and mortality,[3,60–63] shorter postoperative LOS,[62] and higher disease-specific survival.[60–62,64 64] Similarly, HV surgeons have lower postoperative morbidity and mortality than LV surgeons,[4] as well as higher rates of home discharge after surgery (89.1% vs. 81.4%).[63] In an analysis of the National Cancer Database, patients with pancreatic resections performed by HV surgeons had greater 5-year survival rates than patients treated by LV surgeons (15.4% vs. 12.5%, $P < 0.05$), and a 2.26-fold decreased likelihood of perioperative mortality ($P < 0.0001$).[61] The relationship between center and surgeon volume and associated outcomes for pancreatic resection is shown in **Table 4**.

DISPARITIES IN ACCESS TO HIGH VOLUME CARE

Despite the apparent volume–outcome relationship, an overwhelming majority of patients have endocrine surgery by less experienced surgeons,[2,59,65] perhaps due to disparate access to HV care. Treatment by HV centers and surgeons varies greatly by race. Nationally, only 2% of black and 1% of Hispanic patients underwent thyroidectomy by HV surgeons, compared to 7% of white patients,[66] and 13% of Hispanic and 19% of black patients underwent parathyroidectomy by HV surgeons, compared

Table 2
The impact of surgeon and center volume on outcomes after parathyroidectomy

Author, Year	Annual Volume Thresholds	Significant Outcomes
Surgeon volume		
Sosa et al,[31] 1998	• Low: <15 • Medium: 15–49 • High: ≥50	• Complication rates after primary operation were greater for LV surgeons (1.89 vs. 0.91) • Complication rates after reoperation were greater for LV surgeons (3.77 vs. 1.49) • Unadjusted in-hospital mortality rates were greater for LV surgeons (1.00 vs. 0.04)
Stavrakis et al,[28] 2007[a]	• A: 1–3 • B: 4–8 • C: 9–19 • D: 20–50 • E: 51–99 • F: ≥100	• Complication rates were nearly 7-fold higher for group A surgeons than group F surgeons • LOS was longer for lower volume surgeons • Total cost was greater for lower volume surgeons
Al Qurayshi et al,[27] 2017	• Low: 1–2 • Intermediate: 3–19 • High: ≥ 20	• Postoperative complications were more likely for LV surgeons (OR 1.81, 95% CI 1.11–2.97) • Hospital LOS >2 days was more likely for LV surgeons (OR 7.11, 95% CI 3.76–13.45) • Average cost was greater for LV surgeons
Meltzer et al,[29] 2017	• Low: ≤ 20 • High: >40	• Vocal cord paralysis occurred more often in LV surgeons (1.6% vs. 0.2%)
Gray et al,[32] 2022	• Low: <20 • High: >20	• Repeat parathyroid surgery within 1 year of parathyroidectomy was more likely for LV surgeons (OR: 1.63, 95% CI 1.25–2.13) • LOS >2 days was more likely for LV surgeons (OR: 1.22, 95% CI 1.10–1.36) • Surgical complications were more likely for LV surgeons (OR: 1.31, 95% CI 1.01–1.69)
Rajan[33] 2023	• Low: <10 • Medium: 10–30 • High: 31–50 • Very high: >50	• Persistent hypercalcemia occurred more frequently for LV compared to HV surgeons (5.7% vs. 5.1% vs. 5.0% vs. 3.3%); higher surgeon volumes were associated with 13% lower odds of persistent hypercalcemia
Center volume		
Chen et al,[36] 2010	• Low: <50 • High: >50	• Preventable operative failure, based on location of missed parathyroid gland, occurred more frequently at LV centers (89% vs. 13%) • Persistent hyperparathyroidism occurred more often at LV centers (87% vs. 43%)

(*continued on next page*)

Table 2
(continued)

Author, Year	Annual Volume Thresholds	Significant Outcomes
Yeh et al,[37] 2011	• Low: <50 • Medium: 50–99 • High: ≥100	• Persistent hyperparathyroidism was less likely at HV centers (OR 0.42, 95% CI 0.19–0.92)
Abdulla et al,[38] 2015	• Very low: 1–4 • Low: 5–9 • Medium, 10–19 • High: 20–49 • Very high: ≥50	• Total complications occurred more often at very LV centers (6.3% vs. 4.9%) • Surgical complications occurred more often at very LV centers (4.4% vs. 3.5%) • Reoperation rates were higher at very LV centers (6.5% vs. 0.14%)

Abbreviations: HV, high volume; LOS, length of stay; LV, low volume; OR, odds ratio.
[a] This study also includes thyroid and adrenal disease, but analysis is gland-specific.

to 49% of white patients.[67] For benign adrenal disease, only 4% to 5% of Hispanic and 7% to 9% of black patients had surgery by HV surgeons, compared to 78% to 82% of white patients.[43,45] Similarly, patients who underwent pancreatic resection by HV surgeons were more often white (81.1% vs. 74%).[63] Similar trends in racial differences have been reported with respect to access to HV centers.[47,68,69]

Decreased access to HV care leading to treatment delays[70–72] and increased disease severity at the time of surgery[73] likely contributes to the higher complication rates experienced by black patients after surgery compared to white patients.[56,67,74] For parathyroid disease, higher rates of incomplete preoperative imaging assessment have been reported for black patients compared to white patients.[70,75] Thus, decreased access to advanced imaging studies at HV centers may explain the higher percentage of persistent disease in black patients compared to white patients (12.9% vs. 8.4%),[40] though no significant association between race, ethnicity, and reoperation for persistent or recurrent disease has been reported in the literature to date.[37,76] In the management of ACC, limited utilization of HV centers by racial and ethnic minorities may explain the 31% to 32% decreased likelihood of adrenalectomy for ACC for black or Hispanic patients compared to white patients.[77,78] This is important as complete surgical resection offers the only potential for cure.[25] Despite these inequities in ACC treatment, no studies have demonstrated differences in overall survival based on race or ethnicity.[53,77,78]

Although patients from all racial and ethnic groups are increasingly being referred to HV surgeons and centers,[6] this change has occurred at varying degrees depending on race. A comparison of National Inpatient Sample (NIS) data highlights this widening disparity: whereas the percentage of white patients who underwent thyroidectomy by HV surgeons from 2000 to 2004 increased from 1% to 7%, the percentage of black and Hispanic patients treated by HV surgeons only increased from 0.2% to 1.8% and 0% to 1.3%, respectively.

Insurance status may disproportionately impact the ability of select groups to receive HV care. Patients with Medicare, Medicaid, or no insurance had a 1.6-, 1.7-, and 3-fold increased likelihood of thyroidectomy by LV surgeons compared to patients with private insurance, respectively,[79] and a 1.3-, 2.4-, and 3-fold increased likelihood of parathyroidectomy by LV surgeons.[27] For benign adrenal disease, 22% to 30% of Medicare patients, 7% to 8% Medicaid patients, and 2% to 2.4% of uninsured patients had surgery by HV surgeons, compared to 60% to 65% privately insured

Table 3
The impact of surgeon volume on outcomes after adrenalectomy

Author, Year	Annual Volume Thresholds	Significant Outcomes
Gallagher et al,[46] 2007	• ≤1 • 2 • 3–6 • ≥7	• Mean hospital LOS was longer for LV surgeons (7 vs. 6 vs. 7 vs. 5 days)
Park [43] 2009	• Low: <4 • High: ≥4	• Complication rates were higher for LV surgeons (18.3 vs 11.3%) • Mean hospital LOS was longer for LV surgeons (5.5 vs 3.9 days)
Hauch [42] 2015	• Low ≤1 • Intermediate: 2–5 • High: ≥6	• Complication rates were higher for LV surgeons (18.8% vs. 11.6%) • Mean hospital LOS was longer for LV surgeons (4.2 days vs. 2.7 days)
Al-Qurayshi et al,[9] 2016	• Low: ≤1 • Intermediate: 2–6 • High: ≥7	• Complication rates were higher for LV surgeons (39.9% vs. 19.0%) • Prolonged LOS was more likely for LV surgeons (OR 2.65, 95% CI:1.84–3.81) • Average costs were greater for LV surgeons ($16,437.00 vs. $14,772.00 vs. $14,263.00)
Lindeman et al,[44] 2018	• Low: <4 • High: ≥4	• Mortality rates were lower for HV surgeons (0.56% vs. 1.25%) • Complication rates were lower for HV surgeons (10.2% vs. 16.4%); inpatient complications were independently associated with low surgeon volume (OR 0.96, 95% CI: 0.94–0.98)
Anderson et al,[45] 2018	• Low: <6 • High: ≥6	• The likelihood of complications decreased with increasing surgeon volume up to 5.6 cases annually • Mortality rates were higher for LV surgeons (0.6% vs. 2.4%) • Complications were more likely for LV surgeons (OR 1.71, 95% CI: 1.27–2.31) • Prolonged LOS was more likely for LV surgeons (RR 1.46, 95% CI 1.25–1.70) • Higher costs were more likely for LV surgeons (%change: +26.2%, 95% CI 12.6–39.9)

Abbreviations: CI, confidence interval; HV, high volume; LOS, length of stay; LV, low volume; OR, odds ratio; RR risk ratio.

patients.[43,45] At the center level, uninsured patients were 46% to 71% less likely to receive pancreatic resection at a HV center, and Medicaid patients were 40% less likely to have adrenalectomy at HV centers, compared to patients with private insurance.[47,69] For ACC, limited access to HV centers may explain the disproportionate increased utilization of LV centers compared to HV centers by patients with Medicare (38% vs. 24%) compared to patients with private insurance (49% vs. 58%).[52] This has important implications in the management of ACC: as both chemotherapy and surgery are more likely in HV centers,[49,52,53] limited access to HV centers may explain the decreased utilization of chemotherapy for metastatic ACC in patients without private insurance compared to patients with private insurance (54% vs. 64%), and lower rates of surgery for resectable ACC for patients with Medicare (25.7%) or no insurance (4.2%) compared to patients with private insurance (61.1%).[49]

Table 4
The impact of surgeon and center volume on outcomes after pancreatic resection

Author, Year	Annual Volume Thresholds	Significant Outcomes
Surgeon volume		
Eppsteiner et al,[63] 2009	• Low: < 5 • High: ≥ 5	• HV surgeons had a lower adjusted (2.4% vs. 6.4%) • After controlling for patient demographics and factors, HV surgeon was independently associated with a 51% reduction in in-hospital mortality
Schmidt et al,[60] 2010	• Low: < 20 • High: ≥ 20	• HV surgeons performed PD with lower mean blood loss (978 vs. 1788 mL), faster (317 vs. 422 min), and yielded greater lymph node harvest (mean, 13 vs. 9) than LV surgeons • Both groups had equivalent margin status
Wood 2013	• Low: ≤ 12 • High: >12	• Mortality and LOS after PD for HV and LV surgeons at HV centers was not significantly different
Mathur 2015	• Low: ≤ 12 • High: >12	• In-hospital mortality was lower for HV surgeons vs. LV surgeons at HV centers (3% vs. 7%)
Center volume		
Bliss et al,[89] 2014	• Low: < 5 • Medium: 5–18 • High: ≥ 18	• HV centers had lower mortality (3.1% vs. 5.9% vs. 8.1%), fewer complications (33.1% vs. 39.7% vs. 45.8%) and a shorter median LOS (9 vs. 11 vs. 12 days)
Mathur 2015	• Low: ≤ 11 • High: >11	• HV surgeons had similar LOS vs. LV surgeons at HV centers • LOS was significant increased for LV surgeons at LV centers compared to LV surgeons at HV centers. (17 vs. 10 days) • No difference in mortality was observed for LV surgeons at LV hospitals compared to LV surgeons at HV hospitals
Briceno 2017[7]	• Low: < 10 • Medium: 10–20 • High: > 20	• Mortality (30 and 90 days) was higher in LV (5.5%, 10.9%) compared to HV (2.6%, 5.8%) • Patients in LV were less likely to receive neoadjuvant therapy (8.4% vs. 17.3%), obtain R0 resection (72.8% vs. 80.1%) and had lower lymph node harvest (11 vs. 17 nodes)

Abbreviations: HV, high volume; LOS, length of stay; LV, low volume; PD, pancreaticoduodenectomy.

HV surgeons are increasingly clustered to HV centers, which are disproportionately distributed across the United StatesS.[2,5,42,45,59] For example, in 2018, no rural hospitals met Leapfrog minimum volume standard for pancreatectomy[80] which raises concerns regarding the geographic barriers that rural populations may face.[81] Access to HV centers—and by extension, HV surgeons—may depend on patient proximity to teaching hospitals (HV surgeons are more likely located at teaching hospitals),[43,45] urban location (HV surgeons are more likely located in urban areas),[6] or geographic region (HV surgeons are less likely to operate in the Midwest or Southern states).[6] Access to HV centers also depends on patients' financial ability to traverse greater distances.[6] This is seen in thyroid cancer care, which often requires frequent travel to specialized multidisciplinary care centers: privately insured patients and patients from within the highest income-quartile zip codes travel the furthest to receive treatment at HV care centers.[82] The majority of patients who traveled to HV centers for parathyroidectomy were white (92.6%) or privately insured (62.1%).[68] In contrast, racial minorities and patients with Medicare, Medicaid, or no insurance were unlikely to seek a HV parathyroid center if one was not located within 60 miles of their home region.[68] Patients with ACC traveled a median 21.9 miles to academic cancer centers compared to 6.7 miles to community cancer programs[83]; patients from rural areas more frequently had ACC treatment at LV centers compared to HV (2.1% vs. 1.4%, $P < 0.001$).[84] These findings suggest that increased geographic distance may have profound implications on access to HV care, as vulnerable populations may have limited abilities to travel due to physical, geographic, or economic constraints.

SUMMARY

The relationship between surgical volume and outcome is clear. Both surgeon and center volume may serve as proxies for patient- and systems-level factors that have a more direct impact on patient outcomes than volume alone, including improved access to multidisciplinary treatment planning and specialized care, advanced services and technologies, more rigorous disease workup and preoperative optimization, uniform postoperative care processes, and improved postoperative surveillance.[3,85]

Significant disparities following endocrine surgery exist for different racial/ethnic, geographic, and socioeconomic groups. Racial and ethnic minorities and patients of lower socioeconomic status have significantly lower rates of surgery by HV surgeons and centers in comparison to white, non-Hispanic patients and patients of higher socioeconomic status. Disparate access to HV care resulting in decreased utilization of HV centers and lower likelihood of receiving care from a HV surgeon likely contributes to the higher complication rates,[56,67,74,86] worse overall outcomes,[27,67] and prolonged LOS seen in these patients.[5,40,74,87] These outcomes likely also explain the higher costs incurred by racial minorities after surgery.[67,87] The complexities of these disparities require further research to delineate the underlying processes that drive these inequalities. Efforts to identify the patient- and system-level factors required to reduce current inequities in the receipt of high-volume care are needed.

CLINICS CARE POINTS

- Thyroidectomy, parathyroidectomy, adrenalectomy, and surgery for pancreatic neuroendocrine tumors should be performed by HV surgeons to optimize outcomes, including surgical cure.
- Surgery for complex patients (ie, Graves' or thyroid cancer) or rare diseases (ie, ACC) should be performed at HV centers with access to multidisciplinary care teams to mitigate the risk of complications.
- Disparities in access to HV care exists for racial/ethnic minorities and patients of lower socioeconomic status, which may place them at a disproportionate increased risk of complications and recurrent/persistent disease.

DISCLOSURES

The authors of this work have no competing interests to declare and report no proprietary or commercial interest in any product mentioned in this article. This research did not receive any specific grant from funding agencies in the public, commercial, or not-for-profit sector.

REFERENCES

1. Wang TS. Endocrine surgery. Am J Surg 2011;202(3):369–71.
2. Saunders BD, Wainess RM, Dimick JB, et al. Who performs endocrine operations in the United States? Surgery 2003;134(6):924–31.
3. Birkmeyer JD, Siewers AE, Finlayson EV, et al. Hospital volume and surgical mortality in the United States. N Engl J Med 2002;346(15):1128–37.
4. Birkmeyer JD, Stukel TA, Siewers AE, et al. Surgeon volume and operative mortality in the United States. N Engl J Med 2003;349(22):2117–27.
5. Gourin CG, Tufano RP, Forastiere AA, et al. Volume-based trends in thyroid surgery. Arch Otolaryngol Head Neck Surg 2010;136(12):1191–8.
6. Loyo M, Tufano RP, Gourin CG. National trends in thyroid surgery and the effect of volume on short-term outcomes. Laryngoscope 2013;123(8):2056–63.
7. Briceno P, Huston J, Shridhar R, et al. Pancreatic resection at high volume centers improves survival. HPB 2017;19:S171.
8. Erinjeri NJ, Udelsman R. Volume-outcome relationship in parathyroid surgery. best practice & research. Clin Endocrinol Metabol 2019;33(5):101287.
9. Al-Qurayshi Z, Robins R, Buell J, et al. Surgeon volume impact on outcomes and cost of adrenal surgeries. Eur J Surg Oncol 2016;42(10):1483–90.
10. Alsfasser G, Leicht H, Günster C, et al. Volume–outcome relationship in pancreatic surgery. Br J Surg 2015;103(1):136–43.
11. Bedi HK, Jedrzejko N, Nguyen A, et al. Thyroid and parathyroid surgeon case volume influences patient outcomes: a systematic review. Surgical Oncology 2021;38:101550.
12. Kandil E, Noureldine SI, Abbas A, et al. The impact of surgical volume on patient outcomes following thyroid surgery. Surgery 2013;154(6):1346–52 [discussion: 52-3].
13. Lorenz K, Raffaeli M, Barczyński M, et al. Volume, outcomes, and quality standards in thyroid surgery: an evidence-based analysis-European Society of Endocrine Surgeons (ESES) positional statement. Langenbeck's Arch Surg 2020; 405(4):401–25.
14. Melfa G, Porello C, Cocorullo G, et al. Surgeon volume and hospital volume in endocrine neck surgery: how many procedures are needed for reaching a safety level and acceptable costs? A systematic narrative review. G Chir 2018; 39(1):5–11.
15. Schwartz A. Thyroid surgery: who should do it? How should it be done? Thyroid 2005;15(3):185–7.
16. Smith JA, Watkinson JC, Shaha A. Who should perform thyroid surgery? United Kingdom (UK) and United States (US) perspectives with recommendations. Eur Arch Oto-Rhino-Laryngol 2012;269(1):1–4.
17. Swonke ML, Shakibai N, Chaaban MR. Medical malpractice trends in thyroidectomies among general surgeons and otolaryngologists. OTO Open 2020;4(2). https://doi.org/10.1177/2473974x20921141. 2473974X20921141.
18. Kohnen B, Schürmeyer C, Schürmeyer TH, et al. Surgery of benign thyroid disease by ENT/head and neck surgeons and general surgeons: 233 cases of vocal fold paralysis in 3509 patients. Eur Arch Oto-Rhino-Laryngol 2018;275(9): 2397–402.
19. Liang TJ, Liu SI, Mok KT, et al. Associations of volume and thyroidectomy outcomes: a nationwide study with systematic review and meta-analysis. Otolaryngol Head Neck Surg 2016;155(1):65–75.

20. Rubio GA, Koru-Sengul T, Vaghaiwalla TM, et al. Postoperative outcomes in graves' disease patients: results from the nationwide inpatient sample database. Thyroid 2017;27(6):825–31.
21. Kim HI, Kim TH, Choe JH, et al. Surgeon volume and prognosis of patients with advanced papillary thyroid cancer and lateral nodal metastasis. Br J Surg 2018; 105(3):270–8.
22. Sosa JA, Hanna JW, Robinson KA, et al. Increases in thyroid nodule fine-needle aspirations, operations, and diagnoses of thyroid cancer in the United States. Surgery 2013;154(6):1420–6 [discussion: 26-7].
23. Tuggle CT, Roman S, Udelsman R, et al. Same-day thyroidectomy: a review of practice patterns and outcomes for 1,168 procedures in New York State. Ann Surg Oncol 2011;18(4):1035–40.
24. Al-Qurayshi Z, Srivastav S, Kandil E. Comparison of inpatient and outpatient thyroidectomy: demographic and economic disparities. Eur J Surg Oncol 2016; 42(7):1002–8.
25. Patel KN, Yip L, Lubitz CC, et al. The american association of endocrine surgeons guidelines for the definitive surgical management of thyroid disease in adults. Ann Surg 2020;271(3):e21–93.
26. Iacobone M, Scerrino G, Palazzo FF. Parathyroid surgery: an evidence-based volume-outcomes analysis : European Society of Endocrine Surgeons (ESES) positional statement. Langenbeck's Arch Surg 2019;404(8):919–27.
27. Al-Qurayshi Z, Hauch A, Srivastav S, et al. Ethnic and economic disparities effect on management of hyperparathyroidism. Am J Surg 2017;213(6):1134–42.
28. Stavrakis AI, Ituarte PH, Ko CY, et al. Surgeon volume as a predictor of outcomes in inpatient and outpatient endocrine surgery. Surgery 2007;142(6):887–99 [discussion: 87-99].
29. Meltzer C, Klau M, Gurushanthaiah D, et al. Surgeon volume in parathyroid surgery-surgical efficiency, outcomes, and utilization. JAMA Otolaryngol Head Neck Surg 2017;143(8):843–7.
30. Wilhelm SM, Wang TS, Ruan DT, et al. The American association of endocrine surgeons guidelines for definitive management of primary hyperparathyroidism. JAMA Surgery 2016;151(10):959–68.
31. Sosa JA, Powe NR, Levine MA, et al. Profile of a clinical practice: thresholds for surgery and surgical outcomes for patients with primary hyperparathyroidism: a national survey of endocrine surgeons. J Clin Endocrinol Metab 1998;83(8): 2658–65.
32. Gray WK, Navaratnam AV, Day J, et al. Volume-outcome associations for parathyroid surgery in england: analysis of an administrative data set for the getting it right first time program. JAMA Surg 2022;157(7):581–8.
33. Rajan S, Gracie D, Aspinall S. Does surgeon volume impact morbidity following parathyroidectomy? A study of 16,140 parathyroidectomies from the UK registry of endocrine and thyroid surgery (UKRETS) database. World J Surg 2023. https://doi.org/10.1007/s00268-022-06863-9.
34. Neychev VK, Ghanem M, Blackwood SL, et al. Parathyroid surgery can be safely performed in a community hospital by experienced parathyroid surgeons: a retrospective cohort study. Int J Surg 2016;27:72–6.
35. Richmond BK, Eads K, Flaherty S, et al. Complications of thyroidectomy and parathyroidectomy in the rural community hospital setting. Am Surg 2007;73(4): 332–6.

36. Chen H, Wang TS, Yen TWF, et al. Operative failures after parathyroidectomy for hyperparathyroidism: the influence of surgical volume. Ann Surg 2010;252(4): 691–5.
37. Yeh MW, Wiseman JE, Chu SD, et al. Population-level predictors of persistent hyperparathyroidism. Surgery 2011;150(6):1113–9.
38. Abdulla AG, Ituarte PH, Harari A, et al. Trends in the frequency and quality of parathyroid surgery: analysis of 17,082 cases over 10 years. Ann Surg 2015; 261(4):746–50.
39. Donatini G, Marciniak C, Lenne X, et al. Risk factors of redo surgery after unilateral focused parathyroidectomy: conclusions from a comprehensive nationwide database of 13,247 interventions over 6 years. Ann Surg 2020;272(5):801–6.
40. Mitchell J, Milas M, Barbosa G, et al. Avoidable reoperations for thyroid and parathyroid surgery: effect of hospital volume. Surgery 2008;144(6):899–906 [discussion: 06-7].
41. Kazaure HS, Sosa JA. Volume–outcome relationship in adrenal surgery: a review of existing literature. Best Pract Res Clin Endocrinol Metab 2019;33(5):101296.
42. Hauch A, Al-Qurayshi Z, Kandil E. Factors associated with higher risk of complications after adrenal surgery. Ann Surg Oncol 2015;22(1):103–10.
43. Park HS, Roman SA, Sosa JA. Outcomes from 3144 adrenalectomies in the United States: which matters more, surgeon volume or specialty? Arch Surg 2009;144(11):1060–7.
44. Lindeman B, Hashimoto DA, Bababekov YJ, et al. Fifteen years of adrenalectomies: impact of specialty training and operative volume. Surgery 2018; 163(1):150–6.
45. Anderson KL, Thomas SM, Adam MA, et al. Each procedure matters: threshold for surgeon volume to minimize complications and decrease cost associated with adrenalectomy. Surgery 2018;163(1):157–64.
46. Gallagher SF, Wahi M, Haines KL, et al. Trends in adrenalectomy rates, indications, and physician volume: a statewide analysis of 1816 adrenalectomies. Surgery 2007;142(6):1011–21.
47. Simhan J, Smaldone MC, Canter DJ, et al. Trends in regionalization of adrenalectomy to higher volume surgical centers. J Urol 2012;188(2):377–82.
48. Lombardi CP, Raffaelli M, Boniardi M, et al. Adrenocortical carcinoma: effect of hospital volume on patient outcome. Langenbeck's Arch Surg 2012;397(2): 201–7.
49. Tseng J, DiPeri T, Chen Y, et al. Factors associated with non-operative management of resectable adrenocortical carcinoma. J Surg Res 2021;267:651–9.
50. Tseng J, Diperi T, Gonsalves N, et al. Operative approach and case volume are associated with negative resection margins for adrenocortical carcinoma. Surg Endosc 2022;36(12):9288–96.
51. Else T, Kim AC, Sabolch A, et al. Adrenocortical carcinoma. Endocr Rev 2014; 35(2):282–326.
52. MacKinney EC, Holoubek SA, Khokar AM, et al. Treatment differences at high volume centers and low volume centers in non-metastatic and metastatic adrenocortical carcinoma. Am J Surg 2022;223(3):582–6.
53. Gratian L, Pura J, Dinan M, et al. Treatment patterns and outcomes for patients with adrenocortical carcinoma associated with hospital case volume in the United States. Ann Surg Oncol 2014;21(11):3509–14.
54. Grubbs EG, Callender GG, Xing Y, et al. Recurrence of adrenal cortical carcinoma following resection: surgery alone can achieve results equal to surgery plus mitotane. Ann Surg Oncol 2010;17(1):263–70.

55. Gaujoux S, Mihai R. the joint working group of E, Ensat. European Society of Endocrine Surgeons (ESES) and European Network for the Study of Adrenal Tumours (ENSAT) recommendations for the surgical management of adrenocortical carcinoma. BJS (British Journal of Surgery) 2017;104(4):358–76.
56. Holoubek SA, Maxwell J, Fingeret AL. Racial disparities of adrenalectomy. Journal of the Endocrine Society 2020;4(9):bvaa110.
57. Cawich SO, Pearce NW, Naraynsingh V, et al. Whipple's operation with a modified centralization concept: a model in low-volume Caribbean centers. World J Clin Cases 2022;10(22):7620–30.
58. Polonski A, Izbicki JR, Uzunoglu FG. Centralization oF PANCREATIC SURGERY IN EUROpe. J Gastrointest Surg 2019;23(10):2081–92.
59. Acher AW, Weber SM, Pawlik TM. Does the volume-outcome association in pancreas cancer surgery justify regionalization of care? A Review of current controversies. Ann Surg Oncol 2022;29(2):1257–68.
60. Schmidt CM, Turrini O, Parikh P, et al. Effect of hospital volume, surgeon experience, and surgeon volume on patient outcomes after pancreaticoduodenectomy: a single-institution experience. Arch Surg 2010;145(7):634–40.
61. Bilimoria KY, Bentrem DJ, Feinglass JM, et al. Directing surgical quality improvement initiatives: comparison of perioperative mortality and long-term survival for cancer surgery. J Clin Oncol 2008;26(28):4626–33.
62. Kagedan DJ, Goyert N, Li Q, et al. The impact of increasing hospital volume on 90-day postoperative outcomes following pancreaticoduodenectomy. J Gastrointest Surg 2017;21(3):506–15.
63. Eppsteiner RW, Csikesz NG, McPhee JT, et al. Surgeon volume impacts hospital mortality for pancreatic resection. Ann Surg 2009;249(4):635–40.
64. La Torre M, Nigri G, Ferrari L, et al. Hospital volume, margin status, and long-term survival after pancreaticoduodenectomy for pancreatic adenocarcinoma. Am Surg 2012;78(2):225–9.
65. Hauch A, Al-Qurayshi Z, Randolph G, et al. Total thyroidectomy is associated with increased risk of complications for low- and high-volume surgeons. Ann Surg Oncol 2014;21(12):3844–52.
66. Sosa JA, Mehta PJ, Wang TS, et al. Racial disparities in clinical and economic outcomes from thyroidectomy. Ann Surg 2007;246(6):1083.
67. Noureldine SI, Abbas A, Tufano RP, et al. The impact of surgical volume on racial disparity in thyroid and parathyroid surgery. Ann Surg Oncol 2014;21(8):2733–9.
68. Hinson AM, Hohmann SF, Stack BC. Domestic travel and regional migration for parathyroid surgery among patients receiving care at academic medical centers in the United States, 2012-2014. JAMA otolaryngology– head & neck surgery 2016;142(7):641–7.
69. Liu JH, Zingmond DS, McGory ML, et al. Disparities in the utilization of high-volume hospitals for complex surgery. JAMA 2006;296(16):1973–80.
70. Broekhuis JM, Chaves N, Chen HW, et al. Disparities in time to surgeon evaluation among patients with primary hyperparathyroidism. Surgery 2023;173(1):103–10.
71. Mallick R, Xie R, Kirklin JK, et al. Race and gender disparities in access to parathyroidectomy: a need to change processes for diagnosis and referral to surgeons. Ann Surg Oncol 2021;28(1):476–83.
72. Alobuia WM, Meng T, Cisco RM, et al. Racial disparities in the utilization of parathyroidectomy among patients with primary hyperparathyroidism: evidence from a nationwide analysis of Medicare claims. Surgery 2022;171(1):8–16.
73. Kuo LE, Simmons KD, Wachtel H, et al. Racial disparities in initial presentation of benign thyroid disease for resection. Ann Surg Oncol 2016;23(8):2571–6.

74. Hauch A, Al-Qurayshi Z, Kandil E. The effect of race and socioeconomic status on outcomes following adrenal operations. J Surg Oncol 2015;112(8):822–7.
75. Fieber J, Goodsell K, Kelz RR, et al. Racial disparities in primary hyperparathyroidism. World J Surg 2021;45(1):180–7.
76. Kuo LE, Wachtel H, Fraker D, et al. Reoperative parathyroidectomy: who is at risk and what is the risk? J Surg Res 2014;191(2):256–61.
77. Hammad AY, Yen TWF, Carr AA, et al. Disparities in access to care and outcomes in patients with adrenocortical carcinoma. J Surg Res 2017;213:138–46.
78. Holoubek SA, MacKinney EC, Khokar AM, et al. Treatment differences for adrenocortical carcinoma by race and insurance status. J Surg Res 2022;280:169–78.
79. Al-Qurayshi Z, Randolph GW, Srivastav S, et al. Outcomes in endocrine cancer surgery are affected by racial, economic, and healthcare system demographics. Laryngoscope 2016;126(3):775–81.
80. "Complex Adult and Pediatric Surgery: Hospital and Surgeon Volume Fact Sheet 2022." Leapfroggroup.Org, 2022, Available at: ratings.leapfroggroup.org/measure/hospital/complex-adult-and-pediatric-surgery. Accessed Februrary 11, 2023.
81. Dimick JB, Finlayson SR. Rural hospitals and volume standards in surgery. Surgery 2006;140(3):367–71.
82. Greenberg JA, Thiesmeyer JW, Egan CE, et al. Care fragmentation in patients with differentiated thyroid cancer. World J Surg 2022;46(12):3007–16.
83. Stone BV, Tallman JE, Moses KA. Disparate practice patterns and survival outcomes: the impact of centralization of cancer care for adrenocortical carcinoma in the United States. J Urol 2021;206(4):866–72.
84. Kemp Bohan PM, Chang SC, Grunkemeier GL, et al. Impact of mediating and confounding variables on the volume-outcome association in the treatment of pancreatic cancer. Ann Surg Oncol 2023;30(3):1436–48.
85. Gooiker GA, van Gijn W, Wouters MW, et al. Systematic review and meta-analysis of the volume-outcome relationship in pancreatic surgery. Br J Surg 2011;98(4):485–94.
86. Harari A, Li N, Yeh MW. Racial and socioeconomic disparities in presentation and outcomes of well-differentiated thyroid cancer. J Clin Endocrinol Metab 2014;99(1):133–41.
87. Jang S, Mandabach M, Aburjania Z, et al. Racial disparities in the cost of surgical care for parathyroidectomy. J Surg Res 2018;221:216–21.
88. Sosa JA, Bowman HM, Tielsch JM, et al. The importance of surgeon experience for clinical and economic outcomes from thyroidectomy. Ann Surg 1998;228(3):320–30.
89. Bliss LA, Yang CJ, Chau Z, et al. Patient selection and the volume effect in pancreatic surgery: unequal benefits? HPB (Oxford) 2014;16(10):899–906.

Sociodemographic Factors in Pituitary Adenomas

Adriana G. Ioachimescu, MD, PhD

KEYWORDS

• Pituitary adenoma • Elderly • Sex • Race • Ethnicity • Acromegaly
• Socioeconomic status • Transsphenoidal surgery

KEY POINTS

- Pituitary adenomas are increasingly detected in older patients.
- Active surveillance in patients evaluated for transsphenoidal surgery disproportionately occurs in older, Black, Hispanic, uninsured, or government-insured patients.
- Recommendation against surgery and patient refusal of surgery are more prevalent in Black, older and uninsured patients.
- Pituitary surgery at high-volume centers is less likely in patients with Black or Hispanic background, lower socioeconomic status, or uninsured.
- Age, socioeconomic factors, comorbidities, and ethnoracial background have overlapping influences on surgical treatment outcomes.

INTRODUCTION

Pituitary adenomas (PAs) are frequently encountered in adults with a prevalence of 115/100,000. Prolactinomas and nonfunctioning adenomas (NFAs) account for approximately 80% and growth hormone (GH)- and adrenocorticotropic hormone (ACTH)-secreting for 10% to 20%.[1]

According to the Surveillance Epidemiology and End Results (SEER) database, the incidence of PA in the United States increased between 2004 and 2018 from 2.0 $\pm$ 0.12 to 4.67 $\pm$ 0.13/100,000/y. The trend has been attributed to an increase in pituitary incidentalomas, which comprised 42% of PA at the end of the study period.[2] Small nonfunctioning incidentalomas usually do not enlarge or cause health problems, hence are monitored conservatively.[3,4]

PA with suprasellar extension and/or invasion of the surrounding structures can cause mass effects (headaches, vision changes) and anterior hypopituitarism. Recommendation for surgery in NFA is based on the clinical manifestations, tumor size and location. In general, surgery is recommended for GH- and ACTH-secreting

Medical College of Wisconsin, HUB for Collaborative Medicine, Division of Endocrinology, 8701 Watertown Plank Road, Milwaukee, WI 53226, USA
E-mail address: aioachimescu@mcw.edu

Endocrinol Metab Clin N Am 52 (2023) 705–717
https://doi.org/10.1016/j.ecl.2023.05.008
endo.theclinics.com

PA irrespective of tumor size, due to increased morbidity and mortality associated with hormone excess. For prolactin-secreting adenomas, medical treatment with dopamine agonists represents the first-line therapy and surgery is reserved for patients who are resistant or intolerant to medications. Transsphenoidal surgery (TSS) has low rates of surgical morbidity and mortality when performed by experienced neurosurgeons[5–7] and at high-volume centers (HVC) where multidisciplinary care is delivered by experienced clinicians.[8,9] For acromegaly and Cushing's disease, higher biochemical remission rates were demonstrated for dedicated neurosurgeons.[10,11]

Our knowledge about sociodemographic characteristics and their impact on PA presentation and treatment has advanced in recent years. In this article, we discuss the impact of age at diagnosis, sex at birth, racial/ethnic background, socioeconomic status (SES), and insurance type. The aim is to underline current disparities and interactions between sociodemographic factors, with the ultimate goal of designing measures to improve care in vulnerable patients.

AGE AND SEX

Epidemiology

Overall, PA can be diagnosed at any age with predominance in middle-age and elderly adults. A recent SEER analysis found the highest incidence of PA (8.09 ± 0.12) in the age category of 60 to 79 years, which has increased by 29% between 2004 and 2018. Similar with previous literature, the study found a higher PA incidence in women (4.78 ± 0.06) compared to men (3.87 ± 0.05). At the end of the study, there was an increase in PA diagnosis in men (by 7.5%) and a decrease in women (by 5.3%). Of note, prolactinomas only represented 4.7% of tumors in this study[2]; hence, overall PA incidence in women is much higher. The sex/age interaction was explored in an older SEER analysis (2004–2007) which indicated a higher PA incidence at younger ages in women, with more diagnosed after age 50 years.[12]

Clinical characteristics

Age and sex differences have been demonstrated for functional PA.

Prolactinomas disproportionately affect women who often present with microadenomas between ages 25 and 40 years.[13] Conversely, men with prolactinomas usually present with invasive macroadenomas after the age of 40 years. The younger age at diagnosis in women has been attributed to their presentation with galactorrhea and/or oligomenorrhea, which triggers medical evaluation. On the other hand, men with prolactinomas may not seek timely evaluation for manifestations of hypogonadism and often present with mass effect symptoms. However, women with microadenomas rarely experience tumor growth. Some studies showed that tumors in men have higher tumor proliferation markers,[14] and are more likely to be resistant to dopamine agonists than women. Also, rare cases of aggressive prolactinomas requiring surgery, radiation, and even chemotherapy have been described excessively in men.[15] For prolactinomas diagnosed at older ages, fatigue, decreased libido, weakness, and osteoporosis are common manifestations. Radiologically, most tumors diagnosed in this age group are macroprolactinomas which can also present with headaches or vision loss. This has been described in single-institutions series of postmenopausal women[16,17] and men older than 65 years.[18] Finally, one study indicated a third of older men with prolactinomas were incidentally detected.[18] In these reports, most elderly patients responded well to dopamine agonists, biochemically and with tumor shrinkage.

Acromegaly affects both sexes equally, with majority of patients diagnosed at age 40 to 60 years.[19] It has been shown that women with acromegaly are older than men at diagnosis,[19–21] which has been attributed to delay in disease recognition.[22]

Indeed, the opposite effects on estrogen and testosterone on insulin like growth factor 1 (IGF-1) production may cause less obvious physical changes in women than men. Lower IGF-1 levels have been demonstrated in some studies and a meta-analysis.[19–21,23] Larger tumor size at diagnosis was found in women in some studies.[20,21] Women also experience more comorbidities at diagnosis[24]; also, more profound deterioration of their quality of life compared to men.[25] Studies from Finland, Spain, and South Korea found elevated standardized mortality ratio only in women with acromegaly.[26–28] The Spanish study included patients diagnosed with acromegaly at or above age of 65 years and found cardiovascular disease the most common cause of death.[26] This may be related increased prevalence of metabolic syndrome and higher visceral fat accumulation in women with acromegaly compared to men.[29] Surgical remission from single-institution retrospective reports was similar for both sexes,[30] with the exception studies that included a more women than men with invasive tumors.[21]

Cushing's disease affects disproportionately young women who usually present with microadenomas. In an Italian multicenter study (233 women and 47 men), men presented at a younger age with higher urinary free cortisol (UFC) and ACTH levels and a clinical phenotype dominated by bone, muscle and skin involvement.[31] Higher UFC and ACTH levels were confirmed by another study, which also indicated men were at higher risk of hypokalemia, thromboembolic disease, and fractures than women.[32] Although Cushing' s disease is rare in the elderly, a sex disparity was noted in this population, ie, it affects predominantly men presenting with macroadenomas with extrasellar extension.[33]

NFAs affect men and women equally. In population based that do not differentiate between PA types, NFAs are highly represented. A SEER analysis between 2004 and 2007 indicated that median tumor size was larger in men (23 mm) than in women (15 mm).[12]

DISCUSSION

Age and sex differences in functional adenomas are important for PA recognition and treatment. Men and older patients with prolactinoma and Cushing's disease are at higher risk of tumor growth than women. In acromegaly, it is important to consider acromegaly diagnosis in women with a cluster of GH excess manifestations (eg, carpal tunnel syndrome, irregular menstruation, hyperhidrosis) even in absence of characteristic physical changes. Timely diagnosis is important to reduce complications and facilitate timely treatment as GH-secreting tumors have a propensity to grow and become invasive. Cardiovascular risk factors should be treated in elderly patients with acromegaly as they contribute to excess mortality.

Transsphenoidal Surgery in Older Patients

In general, older age and comorbidities increase surgical risk and must be balanced with the benefits of the procedure. A study of the Nationwide Inpatient Sample (NIS) between 1988 and 2005 included 8400 patients older than 65 years; of them, 69.5% were operated at academic hospitals. The inpatient mortality is 3.8%. Patients greater than 80 years old had 30% higher risk of mortality compared to the 65 to 69 year old counterparts.[34] In patients with Cushing's disease age 65 years or older, TSS was associated with an increased risk of adverse outcomes (ie, death and discharge other than home; odds ratio [OR] 20.8) and prolonged hospitalization (OR 2.2). Also in this study, preoperative comorbidities and male gender were associated with adverse outcomes.[35]

A National Cancer Database (NCDB) study of 30,233 patients with PA diagnosed between 2010 and 2015 found that age greater than or equal to 65 years was independently associated with active surveillance (AS) (OR 1.65, 95% CI: 1.48–1.84). Confounding factors were smaller tumor size and closer geographical proximity to the medical center compared to the definitive treatment (DT) group. Academic centers advised DT more often than AS. The main caveat was that tumor functional status and presenting clinical manifestations were not evaluated.[36] Another study from the same database (2004–2015, 34,226 patients) evaluated refusal of surgery, which was encountered in 0.8% cases. Elderly patients were more likely to refuse surgery (OR 2.64); specifically, patients aged 65 years or older accounted for 57% of those who refused surgery and 25% of those who received treatment. The Charlson–Deyo Comorbidity (C/D) Index was however higher in the group who refused surgery. Notably, mortality was higher in patients with macroadenomas who refused surgery.[37]

A recent single-institution study of 908 patients with NFA who underwent TSS between 2007 and 2017 identified 294 of those aged greater than 65 years. There was no difference regarding length of stay, extent of resection, surgical revision for cerebrospinal fluid leak, 30-day readmission, or new hypopituitarism between the young and older groups. Older patients were less likely to experience postoperative vasopressin deficiency but had more hyponatremia compared to young patients.[38]

Another single-institution study (158 NFA patients age 65 years or older and 155 patients age 40–55 years) with TSS between 2008 and 2014 found similar tumor outcomes, ie, gross tumor resection, resolved vision problems, and similar rates of postoperative neurologic complications. Also, postoperative anterior hypopituitarism and vasopressin deficiency were similar between the 2 groups. There were no immediate postoperative deaths. The rate of tumor regrowth in elderly after 32 months was 6.9%, lower compared to the younger group (15.5%).[39]

DISCUSSION

The demographic distribution of PA is currently shifting toward older age, reflecting longer life expectancy and increased use of head imaging. Most PAs in the elderly are NFAs, for which TSS is the primary treatment, and recent studies seem to indicate the procedure is safe. The decision to recommend surgery versus watchful waiting takes into consideration patient-related factors (age, comorbidities) and tumor-specific characteristics (mass effect manifestations, especially vision loss and headaches). If surgery is necessary, patients must undergo a thorough medical clearance and preoperative optimization of comorbidities. Postoperative endocrine complications are usually transient, but require management by an experienced multidisciplinary team, especially in the more complex elderly patient.

RACIAL AND ETHNIC CONSIDERATIONS

Epidemiology

Several population-based studies indicate that incidence of all types of PA is highest in Black patients.[12,40,41] Because of source and methodology of data collection, analyses of clinical and histological types are not available and NFAs are overrepresented. US Central Brain Tumor Registry 2009–2014 reported differences in incidence across racial backgrounds more pronounced with advancing age. Specifically, the incidence rates were 3.8 in Black and 3.15 in White patients ages 15 to 39 years, and 10.5 (Black) and 5.0 (White) after age 40 years.[42] The SEER 2004–2018 study confirmed a higher PA incidence in Blacks (6.72 $\pm$ 0.14) compared to Whites (3.97 $\pm$ 0.04), Asian and Pacific Islanders (3.32 $\pm$ 0.10), and American Indian/Alaska Natives (3.26 $\pm$ 0.26). In addition, Blacks had the highest incidence of pituitary incidentalomas (2.42 ± 0.08) compared to Whites (1.43 ± 0.02) or other racial backgrounds.[2] Another recent NIS study evaluating PA incidence across racial and ethnic categories (1997–2016) confirmed highest rates in Blacks (3.64), followed by Asian/Pacific Islanders (2.57), Hispanics 2.54, and Whites (2.44).[43]

Impact on Presentation

Racial distribution and treatment outcomes for functioning PA have not been studied in nationwide databases. A single-center study at a HVC in US evaluated racial distribution, presentation, and postoperative biochemical results in patients with acromegaly and Cushing's disease. When compared to US Census regional distribution, Black patients with acromegaly and not Cushing's disease were underrepresented. Also, Black patients operated for GH-secreting tumors presented more often with headaches or pituitary incidentalomas than White counterparts and had a higher prevalence of diabetes. Biochemically, IGF-1 level was lower in Black compared to White patients, whereas mean tumor diameter and percentage of tumors with cavernous sinus invasion were similar. There were no differences in biochemical remission postoperatively in the 2 racial groups. In the ACTH-secreting adenoma group, Black patients had a higher proportion of macroadenomas and more preoperative hypopituitarism than White. Postoperative remission rates were borderline higher in White patients, which was statistically associated with higher proportion of macroadenomas.[44]

DISCUSSION

The reason for a higher incidence of PA in Black patients is not known, and genetic and environmental factors have not been studied. Among central nervous system tumors, higher incidence was also observed for meningiomas in the Black population.[12] Incidental detection of PA plays a role; however, it would be expected that many of these tumors were small, which has not been demonstrated. Population-based studies do not provide information regarding clinical presentation or functional PA status. Racial background may matter in acromegaly, with missed or late diagnosis in Black patients. This requires confirmation by larger studies. State and regional registries are necessary to understand the epidemiology, presentation, and prognosis of different types of PA across racial backgrounds and ethnicities.

Influence on Treatment

Surgical treatment, racial and ethnic background for PA overall were evaluated in several US database studies. Similar to other complex procedures, TSS at a HVC has been associated with better outcomes. An NIS study (2008–2012) found lower rates of complications at HVC. Black and Hispanic patients were less likely to be treated at HVC and had higher rates of postoperative complications.[9] In an NIS analysis (1988–2005), there was an increase in the number of patients operated at HVC (defined as 25 or more surgeries/y) at the end of the study period. However, Black, Hispanic and Asians experienced an opposite trend (OR 0.46, 0.28 and 0.49 respectively).[45] Several criteria must be met prior to surgery: clinician recommendation, patient willing to have surgery, and insurance coverage. A SEER/NCDB study (1975–2016) including all PA types other than prolactinomas found that Black and unknown race patients were more likely to be recommended against surgery than White patients (OR 1.13).[46] A NCDB study of 30,233 patients with PA (2010–2015) identified Black race as an independent factor associated with active surveillance (OR 1.12, 95% CI: 1.007–1.23); of note, the tumor type or presenting manifestations were not evaluated.[36] A study from the same database (2004–2015) indicated that Black race was associated with higher odds of refusal of surgery. Notably, mortality was increased in patients with large tumors (diameter >2 cm) who refused surgery. Race other than White/Black was associated with increased survival.[37] A SPARCS (Statewide Planning and Research Cooperative System) database (1995–2015) confirmed that Black patients had lower likelihood to have TSS at HVC and experienced prolonged hospitalization.[47]

Hispanic patients of any race were more likely to undergo TSS at a safety net hospital in Los Angeles rather than at the private hospital. Conversely, non-Hispanic White patients had a higher likelihood to receive care at the private hospital. Of note, both hospitals were affiliated with the same academic institution and surgeries were performed by the same neurosurgeon. No differences were found regarding surgical outcomes.[48]

DISCUSSION

Similar to other surgical fields, disparities in treatment affect minority patients with PA, ie, Black and Hispanic patients are less like to be operated at HVC and benefit from multispecialty care. Cultural differences, language difficulties, and patient transportation are likely contributory factors, and clinician bias requires further study. Many minority patients seek medical advice from local clinicians who may have difficulties to obtain access to higher-level specialized care for their patients.[49] Increased awareness regarding disparities among clinicians, improved patient communication, and establishing bridges between academic institutions and communities can be achieved with targeted educational activities (**Box 1**).

SOCIOECONOMIC DISPARITIES

Disparities steming from low income, food insecurity, and payer status have been well documented in diabetes and obesity. However, their influence on clinical, biochemical, and radiological presentation of PA is largely unknown, especially for GH- and ACTH-secreting types. Several studies explored SES influence on surgical treatment of PA overall or specifically NFA.

A study of the NIS (1997–2016) found an increase in incidence of PA over time in all SES categories.[43] In another study from the same database (1988–2005), higher income patients were more likely to be admitted to HVC for surgical treatment.[45]

Box 1
Influence of age and sex on pituitary adenoma presentation and treatment

- Incidence of overall pituitary adenoma cases in older patients has increased in recent years
- Clinical manifestations of hormone excess in functioning PA are more difficult to recognize in the elderly
- Women diagnosed with growth hormone secreting tumors are slightly older, have lower IGF-1 level, and may experience delayed diagnosis compared to men
- Men with prolactin- and ACTH-secreting tumors have larger tumors compared to women
- Elderly patients are less likely to undergo pituitary surgery in context of active surveillance recommendation and/or patient refusal
- Recent single-institution studies indicate transsphenoidal surgery is safe in the older population

A NCFB study of 30,233 patients with PA diagnosed between 2010 and 2015 indicated that uninsured or government-insured patients were more likely to undergo AS rather than DT (OR 1.58, 95% CI: 1.28–1.94 and 1.45; 95% CI: 1.31–1.61 respectively). Of note, mean tumor size was smaller in the AS group, which is an important confounder. Because of methodology of population-based studies, presenting manifestations or functional tumor status was also not available.[36]

A retrospective review from the University of Southern California Pituitary Center identified 637 patients with NFA who underwent surgery for PA between 2000 and 2021. Lowest tertile zip code level SES was associated with larger tumor size and fewer incidental presentations. Although no significant differences were observed in short-term postoperative complications, postoperative glucocorticoid replacement was more frequently used and complete tumor resection achieved less often compared to highest tertile SES.[50]

Another study from the same institution indicated that patients presenting to a safety net hospital (N = 92) were more often uninsured or had Medicaid compared with patients operated at a private hospital (N = 62). Differences in clinical presentation included more headaches (68.1% vs. 45.7%, $P = 0.0048$), vision loss (63.8% vs. 35.9%, $P < 0.0005$), panhypopituitarism (18.8% vs. 4.3%, $P = 0.0031$), and pituitary apoplexy (18.8% vs. 7.6%, $P = 0.0334$) in the medically underserved populations group. Radiologically, patients in this group presented with larger tumors and more frequent bilateral cavernous sinus invasion than patients with better insurance coverage. The same neurosurgeon operated both groups, and the likelihood of complete tumor resection was similar (73.9% vs. 76.1%). In addition, there were similar rates of improvement in headaches (80% vs. 89%) and vision (82% vs. 84%) postoperatively. The only difference postoperatively was panhypopituitarism (23% vs. 10%, $P = 0.04$), which was attributed to preoperative hormone abnormalities. There were also no differences in long-term outcomes such as tumor recurrence or progression. However, loss to follow-up was seen in 7.6% at the private hospital and 18.6% at the safety net hospital ($P = 0.04$).[48]

A study based on electronic database included patients with PA who underwent endoscopic TSS from 2005 to 2018 at New York-Presbyterian Hospital, Weill Cornell Medicine. Patients with Medicaid insurance (N = 57) were compared with those with non-Medicaid insurance (N = 527). The following parameters were associated with Medicaid insurance: larger tumor diameter, longer postoperative length of stay, higher rate of complications, and long-term cranial neuropathy. There were no differences regarding baseline comorbidities, apoplexy, endocrine outcomes, vision outcomes, or 30-day readmission.[51]

A retrospectively study from University of California San Francisco evaluated 225 patients with NFA who underwent surgery from 2012 to 2019. Higher income was associated with longer postoperative follow-up and lower risk of tumor recurrence. Five factors (race, ethnicity, insurance, primary care physician [PCP] status, and estimated income) affected presentations and outcomes. However, in this study, having a PCP was the single most important variable that was associated with decreased hospital length of stay, readmission, adherence to postoperative care, and lower tumor recurrence.[52]

DISCUSSION

Socioeconomic disparities are associated delayed presentation with larger tumors accompanied by neurological manifestations and hypopituitarism. Surgical outcomes vary across studies and depend on the baseline characteristics of the patient population. Postoperatively, tumor recurrence or progression of tumor residual can occur and radiological surveillance is necessary. Establishing a partnership between pituitary centers and community physicians is important for improved long-term course. Changes in health care policies are necessary to improve access and care of vulnerable populations.

INTERACTIONS BETWEEN ETHNORACIAL CATEGORIES AND SOCIOECONOMIC STATUS

As described above, both ethnoracial background and SES have been associated with lower likelihood of undergoing TSS at HVC (**Table 1**). Interactions between these factors occur, eg, in an NIS study (2008–2012) black and Hispanic patients were more likely to live in the poor income area and have Medicaid insurance.[9] In addition, geographical factors play a role, as reflected by the association between higher neurosurgeon density with admission to an HCV in an NIS study (1988–2005). The same study found that poverty, and not Black or White race, was associated with low likelihood of treatment at an HVC.[45]

Black patients were underrepresented at Emory University in Atlanta, Georgia, in patients with acromegaly, regardless of the SES and travel distance. Such discrepancy was not found in patients with Cushing's disease treated at the same center in the same time period, indicating that disease-specific factors play a role. In patients with acromegaly, the delayed or lack of recognition of pathognomonic features by patients or clinicians may be related to the lower IGF-1 levels. Of note, Black patients with acromegaly had similar short- and long-term biochemical remission rates compared to White patients.[44]

A multihospital academic medical center study from University of Pennsylvania (2013–2019) retrospectively analyzed 46 Black and 46 White patients matched for 29 patient, procedure, and hospital characteristics (American Society of Anesthesiologists grade, Charlson Comorbidity Index, body mass index [BMI], smoking status, etc.). No intergroup differences were found regarding the 90-day readmission, emergency room visits, or unplanned reoperation.[53] On the other hand, the SEER/NCDB study found that Black patients were less likely to be recommended surgery than White patients independent of insurance status, and county (rural or urban) code. The disparity found by this study was also for encountered for glioblastoma, meningioma, and vestibular schwannoma.[46]

Refusal of surgery in patients with macroadenomas disproportionately affected patients in the following groups: age greater than 65 years, Black race, higher C/D index, and government or uninsured status.[37]

A study form the University of North Carolina found that postoperative vasopressin deficiency (diabetes insipidus) occurred more frequently in Hispanic patients who also were more likely to be uninsured.[54]

DISCUSSION

It is known that socioeconomic disparities predominantly affect minority racial and ethnicity population. Targeted health care delivery actions are needed to overcome the obstacles encountered by minority patients. Future studies are warranted to determine whether postoperative racial disparities are mitigated when equal access to specialized centers is attained. Educational activities are important to reduce the implicit bias, increase intercultural communication, and promote meaningful patient–clinician interactions (**Box 2**).

Table 1
Impact of sociodemographic factors on surgical treatment of pituitary adenomas: population-based studies

Study	Database	Patients	PA type	Demographic distribution	Findings
Patil et al,[35] 2007	NIS 1993–2002	3225	ACTH secretory	Women: 81.6% Age >64 y: 4.6%	Older age and male sex had higher risk of adverse outcome.
Mukherjee et al,[45] 2009	NIS 1988–2005	21,717	Not specified	White: 68% Black: 15% Hispanic 10.5% Asian: 3.4% Native American: 0.3% Other: 2.8%	Black, Hispanic, and Asian patients had declining odds of treatment to an HVC over time. Age 25–34 y, household income>$60,000 and more neurosurgeons/100,000 population were associated with HVC treatment.
Goljo et al,[9] 2016	NIS 2008–2012	8812	Not specified	White: 67.2% Black: 18.0% Hispanic: 14.7	Black and Hispanic patients were less likely to be treated at HVC. Black and Hispanic had higher rates of postoperative complications.
McKee et al,[47] 2018	SPARCS 1995–2015	9950	Not specified	White: 56.5% Black: 16.8% Asian: 4.6% Hispanic: 8%	Black patients were less likely to have surgery at HVC. Black patients experienced longer hospitalization.
Birkenbeuel et al,[37] 2022	NCD 2004–2015	32,226	Not specified	Not reported	Black, older, and uninsured (or government insured) patients were more likely to refuse surgery. Black, older, uninsured patients, tumor>2 cm, surgery refusal, and C/D index were associated with increased mortality.
Butterfield et al,[46] 2022	SEER and NCDB 1975–2016	27,506	Other than prolactinoma	Higher incidence in women and Blacks	Black, older, and female patients were less likely to be recommended surgery. Racial disparities were independent on SES and insurance.
Lehrich et al,[36] 2022	NCDB 2010–2015	30,233	Not specified	Age >64 y: 26% Women: 50.6% Black: 19.2%	Black, older, and uninsured patients were less likely to be recommended surgery.

Abbreviations: C/D index, Charlson–Deyo Comorbidity Index; HVC, high-volume center; NCDB, National Cancer Database; NIS, National Inpatient Sample; SEER, Surveillance Epidemiology and End Results; SPARCS, Statewide Planning and Research Cooperative System.

Box 2
Impact of ethnoracial and socioeconomic factors on pituitary adenoma incidence and treatment

- The highest incidence of PA overall is observed in Black patients
- Black, uninsured, or government-insured patients are less likely to be recommended to have pituitary surgery and more likely to refuse surgery
- Patients with low income, uninsured, and Medicaid status have larger tumors and are more often lost to follow-up
- Black and Hispanic patients have a lower likelihood to be operated at high-volume center
- Data on incidence and treatment outcomes according to histological types of PA are not currently available

SUMMARY

Sex and age differences influence presentation and prognosis across PA types. Educational activities targeting an earlier diagnosis can improve patient care. Despite robust epidemiologic evidence of higher PA in Blacks, these patients encounter disparities regarding access to specialized pituitary centers and surgical treatment recommendation. Same pattern was noted for Hispanic, low income, and uninsured or government insured patients with PA. Along with health care policy changes, future research targeting a more granular understanding of inequalities is important to address current shortcomings in patient care.

DISCLOSURES

The author has nothing to disclose.

REFERENCES

1. Melmed S. Pituitary-tumor endocrinopathies. N Engl J Med 2020;382(10):937–50.
2. Watanabe G, Choi SY, Adamson DC. Pituitary incidentalomas in the United States: a national database estimate. World Neurosurg 2022;158:e843–55.
3. Freda PU, Beckers AM, Katznelson L, et al. Pituitary incidentaloma: an endocrine society clinical practice guideline. J Clin Endocrinol Metab 2011;96(4):894–904.
4. Giraldi E, Allen JW, Ioachimescu AG. Pituitary incidentalomas: best practices and looking ahead. Endocr Pract 2023;29(1):60–8.
5. Ciric I, Ragin A, Baumgartner C, et al. Complications of transsphenoidal surgery: results of a national survey, review of the literature, and personal experience. Neurosurgery 1997;40(2):225–36 [discussion: 236-7].
6. Honegger J, Grimm F. The experience with transsphenoidal surgery and its importance to outcomes. Pituitary 2018;21(5):545–55.
7. Barker FG 2nd, Klibanski A, Swearingen B. Transsphenoidal surgery for pituitary tumors in the United States, 1996-2000: mortality, morbidity, and the effects of hospital and surgeon volume. J Clin Endocrinol Metab 2003;88(10):4709–19.
8. Casanueva FF, Barkan AL, Buchfelder M, et al. Criteria for the definition of pituitary tumor centers of excellence (PTCOE): a pituitary society statement. Pituitary 2017;20(5):489–98.
9. Goljo E, Parasher AK, Iloreta AM, et al. Racial, ethnic, and socioeconomic disparities in pituitary surgery outcomes. Laryngoscope 2016;126(4):808–14.

10. Gittoes NJ, Sheppard MC, Johnson AP, et al. Outcome of surgery for acromegaly–the experience of a dedicated pituitary surgeon. QJM 1999;92(12):741–5.
11. Wang YY, Higham C, Kearney T, et al. Acromegaly surgery in Manchester revisited–the impact of reducing surgeon numbers and the 2010 consensus guidelines for disease remission. Clin Endocrinol 2012;76(3):399–406.
12. McDowell BD, Wallace RB, Carnahan RM, et al. Demographic differences in incidence for pituitary adenoma. Pituitary 2011;14(1):23–30.
13. Mindermann T, Wilson CB. Age-related and gender-related occurrence of pituitary adenomas. Clin Endocrinol 1994;41(3):359–64.
14. Fainstein Day P, Glerean M, Lovazzano S, et al. Gender differences in macroprolactinomas: study of clinical features, outcome of patients and ki-67 expression in tumor tissue. Front Horm Res 2010;38:50–8.
15. Trouillas J, Delgrange E, Wierinckx A, et al. Clinical, pathological, and molecular factors of aggressiveness in lactotroph tumours. Neuroendocrinology 2019;109(1):70–6.
16. Santharam S, Tampourlou M, Arlt W, et al. Prolactinomas diagnosed in the postmenopausal period: clinical phenotype and outcomes. Clin Endocrinol 2017;87(5):508–14.
17. Shimon I, Bronstein MD, Shapiro J, et al. Women with prolactinomas presented at the postmenopausal period. Endocrine 2014;47(3):889–94.
18. Shimon I, Hirsch D, Tsvetov G, et al. Hyperprolactinemia diagnosis in elderly men: a cohort of 28 patients over 65 years. Endocrine 2019;65(3):656–61.
19. Dal J, Skov BG, Andersen M, et al. Sex differences in acromegaly at diagnosis: a nationwide cohort study and meta-analysis of the literature. Clin Endocrinol 2021;94(4):625–35.
20. Ioachimescu AG, Handa T, Goswami N, et al. Gender differences and temporal trends over two decades in acromegaly: a single center study in 112 patients. Endocrine 2020;67(2):423–32.
21. Park SH, Ku CR, Moon JH, et al. Age- and sex-specific differences as predictors of surgical remission among patients with acromegaly. J Clin Endocrinol Metab 2018;103(3):909–16.
22. Kreitschmann-Andermahr I, Siegel S, Kleist B, et al. Diagnosis and management of acromegaly: the patient's perspective. Pituitary 2016;19(3):268–76.
23. Parkinson C, Ryder WD, Trainer PJ, et al. The relationship between serum GH and serum IGF-I in acromegaly is gender-specific. J Clin Endocrinol Metab 2001;86(11):5240–4.
24. Esposito D, Ragnarsson O, Johannsson G, et al. Prolonged diagnostic delay in acromegaly is associated with increased morbidity and mortality. Eur J Endocrinol 2020;182(6):523–31.
25. Ballesteros-Herrera D, Briseno-Hernandez P, Perez-Esparza R, et al. Differences in quality of life between genders in acromegaly. Endocrinol Diabetes Metab 2021;4(2):e00229.
26. Biagetti B, Iglesias P, Villar-Taibo R, et al. Mortality in acromegaly diagnosed in the elderly in Spain is higher in women compared to the general Spanish population. J Clin Endocrinol Metab 2023. https://doi.org/10.1210/clinem/dgad141.
27. Park KH, Lee EJ, Seo GH, et al. Risk for acromegaly-related comorbidities by sex in korean acromegaly. J Clin Endocrinol Metab 2020;105(4). https://doi.org/10.1210/clinem/dgz317.
28. Ritvonen E, Loyttyniemi E, Jaatinen P, et al. Mortality in acromegaly: a 20-year follow-up study. Endocr Relat Cancer 2016;23(6):469–80.

29. Ciresi A, Amato MC, Pivonello R, et al. The metabolic profile in active acromegaly is gender-specific. J Clin Endocrinol Metab 2013;98(1):E51–9.
30. Agrawal N, Ioachimescu AG. Prognostic factors of biochemical remission after transsphenoidal surgery for acromegaly: a structured review. Pituitary 2020; 23(5):582–94.
31. Pecori Giraldi F, Moro M, Cavagnini F. Study Group on the Hypothalamo-Pituitary-Adrenal Axis of the Italian Society of E. Gender-related differences in the presentation and course of Cushing's disease. J Clin Endocrinol Metab 2003;88(4): 1554–8.
32. Zilio M, Barbot M, Ceccato F, et al. Diagnosis and complications of Cushing's disease: gender-related differences. Clin Endocrinol 2014;80(3):403–10.
33. Amodru V, Ferriere A, Tabarin A, et al. Cushing's Syndrome in the elderly: data from the european registry on cushing's syndrome. Eur J Endocrinol 2023. https://doi.org/10.1093/ejendo/lvad008.
34. Grossman R, Mukherjee D, Chaichana KL, et al. Complications and death among elderly patients undergoing pituitary tumour surgery. Clin Endocrinol 2010;73(3): 361–8.
35. Patil CG, Lad SP, Harsh GR, et al. National trends, complications, and outcomes following transsphenoidal surgery for Cushing's disease from 1993 to 2002. Neurosurg Focus 2007;23(3):E7.
36. Lehrich BM, Birkenbeuel JL, Roman K, et al. Treatment selection towards active surveillance over definitive treatment for pituitary adenomas is influenced by sociodemographic factors. Clin Neurol Neurosurg 2022;222:107455.
37. Birkenbeuel JL, Lehrich BM, Goshtasbi K, et al. Refusal of surgery in pituitary adenoma patients: a population-based analysis. Cancers 2022;14(21). https://doi.org/10.3390/cancers14215348.
38. Pereira MP, Oh T, Joshi RS, et al. Clinical characteristics and outcomes in elderly patients undergoing transsphenoidal surgery for nonfunctioning pituitary adenoma. Neurosurg Focus 2020;49(4):E19.
39. Zhan R, Ma Z, Wang D, et al. Pure endoscopic endonasal transsphenoidal approach for nonfunctioning pituitary adenomas in the elderly: surgical outcomes and complications in 158 patients. World Neurosurg 2015;84(6):1572–8.
40. Heshmat MY, Kovi J, Simpson C, et al. Neoplasms of the central nervous system. incidence and population selectivity in the Washington DC, metropolitan area. Cancer 1976;38(5):2135–42.
41. Fan KJ, Pezeshkpour GH. Ethnic distribution of primary central nervous system tumors in Washington, DC, 1971 to 1985. J Natl Med Assoc 1992;84(10):858–63.
42. Gittleman H, Cote DJ, Ostrom QT, et al. Do race and age vary in non-malignant central nervous system tumor incidences in the United States? J Neuro Oncol 2017;134(2):269–77.
43. Ghaffari-Rafi A, Mehdizadeh R, Ghaffari-Rafi S, et al. Demographic and socioeconomic disparities of pituitary adenomas and carcinomas in the United States. J Clin Neurosci 2022;98:96–103.
44. Ioachimescu AG, Goswami N, Handa T, et al. Racial disparities in acromegaly and cushing's disease: a referral center study in 241 patients. J Endocr Soc 2022;6(1):bvab176.
45. Mukherjee D, Zaidi HA, Kosztowski T, et al. Predictors of access to pituitary tumor resection in the United States, 1988-2005. Eur J Endocrinol 2009;161(2):259–65.
46. Butterfield JT, Golzarian S, Johnson R, et al. Racial disparities in recommendations for surgical resection of primary brain tumours: a registry-based cohort analysis. Lancet 2022;400(10368):2063–73.

47. McKee S, Yang A, Kidwai S, et al. The socioeconomic determinants for transsphenoidal pituitary surgery: a review of New York State from 1995 to 2015. Int Forum Allergy Rhinol 2018;8(10):1145–56.
48. Cyprich J, Pangal DJ, Rutkowski M, et al. Comparative preoperative characteristics and postoperative outcomes at a private versus a safety-net hospital following endoscopic endonasal transsphenoidal resection of pituitary adenomas. J Neurosurg 2020;134(3):742–9.
49. Bach PB, Pham HH, Schrag D, et al. Primary care physicians who treat blacks and whites. N Engl J Med 2004;351(6):575–84.
50. Cote DJ, Ruzevick JJ, Kang KM, et al. Association between socioeconomic status and presenting characteristics and extent of disease in patients with surgically resected nonfunctioning pituitary adenoma. J Neurosurg 2022;137(6):1699–706.
51. Younus I, Gerges M, Schwartz TH, et al. Impact of Medicaid insurance on outcomes following endoscopic transsphenoidal pituitary surgery. J Neurosurg 2020;134(3):801–6.
52. Osorio RC, Pereira MP, Joshi RS, et al. Socioeconomic predictors of case presentations and outcomes in 225 nonfunctional pituitary adenoma resections. J Neurosurg 2021;1–12. https://doi.org/10.3171/2021.4.JNS21907.
53. Haldar D, Glauser G, Winter E, et al. The influence of race on outcomes following pituitary tumor resection. Clin Neurol Neurosurg 2021;203:106558.
54. Tiwari C, Maung E, Gelinne A, et al. Disparities in postoperative endocrine outcomes after endoscopic-assisted transsphenoidal pituitary adenoma resection. Cureus 2022;14(11):e31934.

Hormonal Injustice

Environmental Toxicants as Drivers of Endocrine Health Disparities

Margaret C. Weiss, BS[a,b,c,1], Luyu Wang, BS[b,c,1],
Robert M. Sargis, MD, PhD[b,c,d,e,*]

KEYWORDS

- Disparities • Endocrine-disrupting chemicals • Environmental justice
- Endocrine health • Diabetes • Obesity • Thyroid • Reproductive

KEY POINTS

- Vulnerable populations carry a disproportionate burden of multiple endocrine disorders and their associated comorbidities and medical costs.
- Racial/ethnic minorities, those with low incomes, and other disadvantaged groups are disproportionately exposed to various endocrine-disrupting chemicals (EDCs) linked to adverse endocrine health effects.
- Achieving endocrine health equity requires comprehensive efforts to eliminate environmental injustice.

INTRODUCTION

A wide spectrum of endocrine disorders are characterized by health disparities, including metabolic,[1] thyroid,[2] and reproductive disorders.[3] Although metabolic disease prevalence has increased across sociodemographic groups, minority racial/ethnic groups carry a greater disease burden.[4] This difference is exacerbated by educational and socioeconomic disparities,[5] reduced access to resources, and systemic oppression.[6] Evidence indicates that vulnerable populations are disproportionately exposed to various environmental toxicants, including multiple endocrine-disrupting chemicals

[a] School of Public Health, University of Illinois at Chicago, 1603 West Taylor Street, Chicago, IL 60612, USA; [b] College of Medicine, University of Illinois at Chicago, 1853 West Polk Street, Chicago, IL 60612, USA; [c] Division of Endocrinology, Diabetes, and Metabolism, University of Illinois at Chicago, 835 South Wolcott, Suite E625, M/C 640, Chicago, IL 60612, USA; [d] Chicago Center for Health and Environment, School of Public Health, University of Illinois at Chicago, 1603 West Taylor Street, Chicago, IL 60612, USA; [e] Section of Endocrinology, Diabetes, and Metabolism, Jesse Brown Veterans Affairs Medical Center, 820 South Damen, Chicago, IL 60612, USA
[1] These authors contributed equally to this work.
* Corresponding author. Division of Endocrinology, Diabetes, and Metabolism, University of Illinois at Chicago, 835 South Wolcott, Suite E625, M/C 640, Chicago, IL 60612.
E-mail address: rsargis@uic.edu

Endocrinol Metab Clin N Am 52 (2023) 719–736
https://doi.org/10.1016/j.ecl.2023.05.009
0889-8529/23/Published by Elsevier Inc.

(EDCs).[7] An analysis of EDC exposures and disease burden across racial/ethnic groups noted higher exposures among non-Hispanic Blacks and Mexican Americans relative to non-Hispanic Whites.[8] Furthermore, per capita EDC-associated health care costs are higher among people of color. Of $340 billion in US health care costs associated with EDCs, Black and Mexican American communities accounted for 31.4% of total expenditures while only comprising 26.1% of the population.[8] The disproportionate burden of hazardous chemical exposures borne by vulnerable communities is an environmental justice crisis with multigenerational consequences.[9] This review highlights key data linking EDC exposures to endocrine health disparities.

HEALTH DISPARITIES IN ENDOCRINOLOGY

Metabolic Disorders

Projected to afflict 783 million adults by 2045, global diabetes prevalence has increased dramatically over recent decades.[10] In the United States alone, 37.3 million people have diabetes; however, the disease burden is not uniform.[11] Diabetes prevalence is markedly lower among non-Hispanic Whites compared with all other minority racial/ethnic groups. Critically, racial/ethnic minorities also suffer from higher diabetes-associated morbidity and mortality.[12] Marked diabetes disparities are also noted by socioeconomic status (SES).[13]

In 2017, US adult obesity prevalence reached an astonishing 41.9%.[14] Prevalence was highest among Hispanics/Latinos and non-Hispanic Blacks. Across all groups, prevalence increases with lower educational attainment. Although associations between obesity rates and SES remain somewhat murky, SES seems to predict body fat distribution, with those of lower SES accumulating fat more centrally, a characteristic associated with various metabolic comorbidities.[13] Drivers of obesity disparities include differences in food availability arising from variations in the retail food environment that concentrate poor-quality resources in more disadvantaged areas,[15] and neighborhood insecurity and a lack of green spaces[16]; more recently, chemical exposures have been implicated.[17]

Nonalcoholic fatty liver disease (NAFLD) is a metabolic disorder characterized by alcohol-independent hepatic fat accumulation associated with inflammation, fibrosis, cirrhosis, liver failure, and hepatocellular carcinoma. By 2030, approximately 100.9 million US adults are projected to be afflicted by NAFLD.[18] Importantly, NAFLD prevalence and complications exhibit notable disparities, with the greatest disease burden among Hispanics/Latinos.[19] Although men are disproportionately affected, evidence indicates that women may have higher rates of NAFLD-related complications.[20] NAFLD disparities are also noted based on SES, with low-income populations experiencing greater prevalence, disease progression, and complications.[21]

Thyroid Disorders

Globally, 200 million people are affected by thyroid diseases,[22] with incidence increasing with age, iodine deficiency, and radiation exposure.[23] Thyroid nodules are more prevalent in women than men, with White individuals disproportionately affected.[24] Importantly, epidemiologic evidence links thyroid nodules with the metabolic syndrome. While this association is observed in both sexes, women are at greater risk of developing thyroid nodules than men with the same metabolic disturbances.[25] Although diagnostic bias may confound the associations, thyroid cancer is more prevalent among Whites, with socioeconomic factors predicting survival.[25,26] Despite this, evidence suggests that Black patients have lower survival rates regardless of screening or SES.[27] In addition to disparities in thyroid cancer, Blacks are more likely to develop thyrotoxicosis than Whites,[28] with disparities also present for hypothyroidism. Among those with subclinical hypothyroidism and comorbid congestive heart failure, Blacks have higher mortality rates than non-Blacks.[29]

Reproductive Disorders

Racial/ethnic and socioeconomic disparities characterize women's health from menarche to menopause. For example, Hispanic/Latina and Black individuals reach menarche at younger ages than their White counterparts.[30] Furthermore, early onset of menarche is associated with fibroid tumors and increased risk for breast and ovarian cancer.[31] Among women with fibroids, racial minorities with lower SES had greater fibroid severity and decreased health-related quality of life.[32] In addition to earlier menarche, Black women reach menopause earlier than White women, and they experience longer menopausal transitions.[33] Polycystic ovarian syndrome (PCOS) is an endocrine disorder characterized by ovarian cysts, menstrual irregularities, hyperandrogenism, infertility, and metabolic dysfunction. Women of lower SES are at greater risk of developing PCOS, and Black women with PCOS are more likely to develop metabolic complications.[34]

Among men, reproductive disparities are also notable. Compared with Whites, Black individuals were significantly more likely to have lower sperm volume and concentration with fewer motile sperm.[35] These issues are likely exacerbated by the fact that Black populations are disproportionately burdened by metabolic disorders, which also negatively affect spermatogenic activity and semen quality.[36]

Adrenal Disorders

Disruptions in adrenal function adversely affect health and development in myriad ways. Compared with White men, Black men are more likely to exhibit dysregulated cortisol secretion patterns, which are linked to multiple adverse health outcomes.[37] Furthermore, conditions of excess cortisol production are more prevalent among women.[38] Primary hyperaldosteronism, the most common cause of secondary hypertension, is more common in Black populations.[39] Androgen excess is linked to PCOS and other reproductive disorders in men and women, with prevalence varying by race/ethnicity and SES. Collectively, the available evidence points to race/ethnicity-, gender-, and income-based disparities across a spectrum of endocrine disorders; achieving health equity requires identifying and addressing the drivers of these differences.

ENDOCRINE-DISRUPTING CHEMICAL EXPOSURE DISPARITIES

Although various social and structural determinants of health contribute to disparities in endocrine health, less appreciated are the contributions of differential exposures to EDCs. The Endocrine Society defines EDCs as "an exogenous chemical, or mixture of chemicals, that can interfere with any aspect of hormone action." More than 500 EDCs have been identified, including polychlorinated biphenyls (PCBs), bisphenols, phthalates, organochlorine (OC) pesticides, per/polyfluoroalkyl substances (PFASs), metals/metalloids, flame retardants, and air pollutants, among others. Critically, exposure to these chemicals is not uniform across populations. Rather certain groups are disproportionately exposed, including various minority racial/ethnic groups, with noted gender-based disparities.[8,40,41] Those with low incomes or of lower SES are also disproportionately exposed.[42] These exposure disparities are driven by multiple social factors, including dietary patterns, consumer product usage, living conditions, labor practices, and geography,[41] all of which are driven by current and historical policies influenced by racist and classist power structures. Thus, environmental injustice drives exposure disparities. The following highlights key literature regarding notable EDC exposure disparities and adverse endocrine health effects (**Fig. 1**, **Table 1**).

Polychlorinated Biphenyls

PCBs are a class of persistent organic pollutants (POPs) historically used for a multitude of industrial applications. Although PCB production was banned in the US in 1979, they persist in the environment because of their long half-lives and continued leaching from older consumer products and industrial waste facilities. Their hydrophobicity and chemical stability results in accumulation in the fatty tissue of animals over time through consumption of contaminated food or prey, resulting in biomagnification at higher trophic levels of the food system. Consequently, human exposure continues through air, soil, food, and water sources. Following exposure, PCBs are associated with multiple adverse endocrine health effects. PCBs mimic the structure of thyroxine and interfere with thyroid hormone homeostasis.[43] PCBs are also associated with metabolic dysfunction in human studies.[44,45] Specifically, a 2014 meta-analysis revealed that individuals exposed to the highest levels of PCBs had a two-fold higher risk of diabetes.[46] In cellular and animal models, PCBs alter insulin release and insulin sensitivity, among other effects, resulting in a diabetic phenotype.[47] Both epidemiologic and preclinical data also link PCBs with NAFLD.[48]

PCB exposure is not homogenous across racial/ethnic groups. Among US adults, Black individuals have significantly higher blood PCB levels than all other racial/ethnic groups, whereas among adolescents and young adults, Pacific Islanders and Native Americans have the highest levels.[49] This disparity may be particularly important in

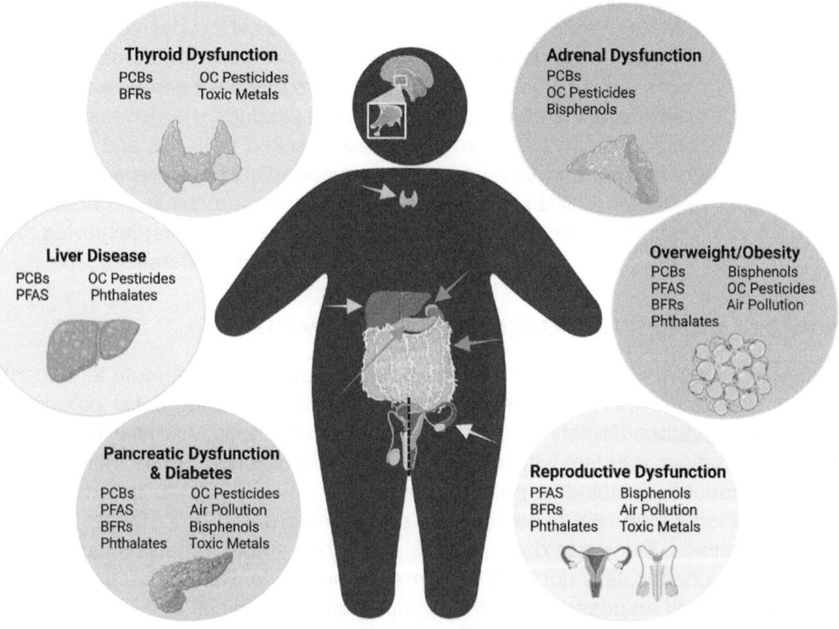

Fig. 1. Summary of endocrine-disrupting chemicals with known exposure disparities and their effects on the endocrine system. These manifestations may be direct effects or downstream consequences of hypothalamic and/or pituitary dysfunction. BFRs, brominated flame retardants; OC Pesticides, organochlorine pesticides; PCBs, polychlorinated biphenyls; PFAS, per/polyfluoroalkyl substances. (*Created with* BioRender.com.)

Table 1
Endocrine-disrupting chemical exposure disparities

Endocrine Disruptor	More Highly Exposed Groups	Endocrine Impacts
Polychlorinated biphenyls	Non-Hispanic Black populations[49] Pacific Islanders and Native Americans[49] US-born individuals[50] Immigrant women[119] Low income[51]	Thyroid dysfunction[43] Obesity[44] Diabetes[45,47] Adrenal dysfunction[10,58] NAFLD[48]
Phthalates	Women[60] Non-Hispanic Black populations[59] Mexican Americans[59] Low income[61]	Male infertility[56] Diabetes[43,44] Obesity[129,130]
Bisphenols	Women[67] Low income[67,70,71] Non-Hispanic Black populations[68,69]	Polycystic ovarian syndrome[65] Male infertility[56] Obesity[44] Diabetes[66] Adrenal dysfunction[58]
Organochlorine pesticides	Non-Hispanic Black populations[83] Asian populations[84] Women[84] Immigrants[7,50] Low income[85]	Thyroid dysfunction[75–77] Diabetes[46,80,81] Obesity[81,82] Adrenal dysfunction[58] NAFLD[131]
Air pollution	Non-Hispanic Black populations[93,94] Hispanic/Latinx Americans[97] Low income[93,94,98,99]	Diabetes[86,87] Obesity[88,89] Infertility[91,92]
Per- and polyfluoroalkyl substances	Women[103] Chinese populations[104] Black populations[102] Hispanic/Latinx populations[102] Low income[103,105]	Diabetes[100] Obesity[100] Reproductive dysfunction[100] NAFLD[101]
Toxic metals	Black populations[116,117] Hispanic/Latinx Americans[116,118] Low income[116,120] Immigrants[119]	Diabetes[111,132] Reproductive dysfunction[113] Infertility[114] Thyroid dysfunction[115]
Brominated flame retardants	Low income[124,125] Women[122] Non-Hispanic Black populations[126] Hispanic/Latinx populations[126]	Diabetes[123] Obesity[123] Thyroid dysfunction[123] Reproductive dysfunction[123]

the United States where PCB levels are generally higher in US-born individuals than immigrants.[50] It is postulated that these PCB exposure patterns are primarily driven by dietary consumption and past exposures, but more evidence is needed.[49] Lastly, occupation and housing are associated with higher PCB levels, and there are noted income-based disparities as well.[51,52]

Phthalates

Phthalates are a family of nonpersistent phthalic acid esters with short half-lives but numerous exposure sources. Often classified by their molecular weight, low-molecular-weight phthalates are commonly used in personal care products and solvents, whereas high-molecular-weight phthalates serve as plasticizers in medical equipment and food packaging.[53] These compounds leach from products, leading to exposure via ingestion, dermal contact, or inhalation.

Although phthalates are nonpersistent pollutants, continuous and repeated exposure can promote adverse health effects. In women, phthalates are associated with ovarian and uterine dysfunction, contributing to the development of PCOS, uterine fibroids, and endometriosis through direct estrogenic effects.[54] During pregnancy, maternal phthalate exposure is associated with placental disruption, pregnancy loss, and greater risk of preterm birth.[55] Phthalates also disrupt male sex steroid signaling, including antagonism of androgen receptor signaling. Consequently, phthalates are linked to hypospadias and male infertility.[56] Moreover, via interactions with various nuclear receptors, phthalates promote diabetogenic and obesogenic effects.[43,44] Indeed, numerous epidemiologic studies associate phthalates and phthalate metabolites with increased diabetes risk.[57] Lastly, phthalates disrupt enzymes involved in adrenal hormone production.[58]

Women are disproportionately expose to phthalates, likely a consequence of their greater use of personal care products. Among women, Black and Mexican American women have higher levels of almost all phthalates and phthalate metabolites.[59] This may be the case because beauty products directly marketed to women of color contain higher levels of phthalates and other chemicals.[60] Marketing strategies perpetuate European beauty standards among minority populations, leading to disproportionate use of skin lighteners, hair relaxers/straighteners, and odor reduction products known to contain EDCs.[60] Similarly, inexpensive building materials, fast food, and consumer products are more likely to contain a variety of EDCs, including phthalates, placing those of low SES at greater risk of exposure.[61,62]

Bisphenols

Bisphenols, such as bisphenol A (BPA), are found in numerous consumer products, including the linings of food containers, plastics, thermal paper, and preservatives.[63] Like phthalates, bisphenols are nonpersistent pollutants; however, humans are continuously exposed. BPA is a well-studied EDC that disrupts multiple signaling cascades, including estrogen receptors, growth factor receptors, and other pathways implicated in diabetes, cardiovascular disease, and cancer.[64] As a xenoestrogen, BPA is linked to multiple reproductive disorders, including PCOS, cryptorchidism, and male infertility.[56,65] Because of BPA's disruption of metabolic pathways, human and preclinical studies have linked BPA exposure with increased metabolic disease risk, including obesity and diabetes.[44,66] The latter findings are supported by robust in vivo and in vitro data demonstrating BPA's capacity to perturb metabolic homeostasis.[64] Additionally, BPA is implicated in adrenal dysfunction through targeting of enzymes involved in the synthesis of glucocorticoids, mineralocorticoids, and androgens.[58]

Across the general population, women and those with lower incomes have greater BPA exposure.[67] Women of color, especially Black women in the United States, have higher BPA levels.[68,69] Furthermore, low-income families and those that received emergency food assistance have higher levels of BPA independent of other sociodemographic factors.[70,71]

Organochlorine Pesticides

Historically used throughout the world, OC pesticides are POPs that were banned in the United States in the 1970s. Despite their toxicity, several OC pesticides are still used in developing countries, including dichlorodiphenyltrichloroethane (DDT), hexachlorocyclohexane, aldrin, and dieldrin.[72] Because of their persistence and biomagnification, OC pesticides continue to contaminate soil, water, air, and fatty meat and fish.[73] US biomonitoring data indicate near universal exposure to OC pesticides, such as DDT and its metabolites.[74]

Many studies have linked OC pesticides with endocrine dysfunction, including disruptions in thyroid hormone function and an increased risk of thyroid cancer.[75–77] OC pesticides are also associated with other endocrine-related cancers, including prostate and breast.[78,79] Levels of multiple OC pesticides are associated with diabetes and obesity.[46,80–82] Lastly, because of its lipophilicity, DDT accumulates in adrenal glands.[58]

Prospective studies show that OC pesticide levels are higher among Black and Asian women compared with White women.[83,84] Furthermore, recently immigrated Hispanics/Latinos have higher levels of OC pesticides than longer-term US residents of the same race/ethnicity, suggesting important international exposure disparities.[7,50] Importantly, OC pesticide exposures vary based on occupation and income, with agricultural work an important exposure source.[85]

Air Pollutants

Air pollution includes atmospheric contamination by a wide array of chemical, biologic, and physical agents. The most common air pollutants include fine particulate matter less than 10 μm and less than 2.5 μm in size (PM_{10} and $PM_{2.5}$, respectively), ozone, and nitrogen dioxide (NO_2), among others. Although outdoor air pollution is more widely appreciated, indoor air pollution is increasingly recognized to adversely impact health. Many studies have linked various air pollutants to endocrine disorders. Indeed, elevated PM and NO_2 exposures are associated with dysregulated glucose homeostasis and increased diabetes risk.[86,87] Additionally, air pollution is implicated in the progression of childhood and adult obesity.[88,89] This metabolic dysfunction is likely further exacerbated by associations between PM and other conditions, such as chronic liver disease.[90] Lastly, although more evidence is needed, air pollution has been linked to male infertility, including reduced sperm motility and impaired gametogenesis.[91,92]

Critically, air quality varies geographically. Minority communities are disproportionately situated in areas with higher levels of multiple air pollutants, with exposures amplified by low-income status.[93,94] Additionally, minority communities are more likely to live in geographic areas with higher levels of traffic-related air pollution, which contributes significantly to NO_2 exposure and more toxic forms of PM.[95,96] Black and Hispanic/Latino communities have been noted to have some of the highest air pollution exposures.[97] With the implementation of federal environmental policies, absolute air quality in the US has improved since 1990; however, racial/ethnic exposure disparities persist under the influence of income inequality and historical discriminatory policies.[7,98] Moreover, lower income status is consistently shown to predict exposure to higher air pollution levels independent of race, ethnicity, or sex.[99]

Per- and Polyfluoroalkyl Substances

PFASs encompass a diverse family of synthetic chemicals widely used in manufacturing and consumer products, including food packaging, cookware, and outerwear among others. Considered "forever chemicals," PFASs are another class of POPs with long half-lives that contaminate food, water, soil, and air. Various PFASs are associated with multiple adverse endocrine effects. These include links to diabetes, obesity, NAFLD, and reproductive dysfunction.[100,101]

Importantly, PFAS exposures vary across populations. Black and Hispanic/Latino populations have been noted to have significantly higher PFAS levels compared with Whites.[102,103] Although some studies suggest that PFAS levels have begun to decline, this is not true across all racial/ethnic groups. For example, individuals of Chinese descent were found to have almost no decline in PFAS levels between 1999 and 2011.[104] Beyond race/ethnicity, lower SES and food insecurity are also linked to PFAS exposures, potentially as a consequence of food packaging and chemicals in less expensive personal care products.[103,105] A recent report by the National Academies recommends PFAS testing in those likely to have a history of elevated exposures, including those based on occupation and place of residence.[106] Such expanded testing may further illuminate PFAS exposure disparities.

Toxic Metals/Metalloids

Toxic metal/metalloid exposures include organic and inorganic forms of several elements, including arsenic, cadmium, and lead. These elements leach naturally into groundwater via geochemical processes; however, environmental exposures are enhanced via historical and current anthropogenic activities. Climate change also increases exposure to toxic metals/metalloids. Arsenic exposure threatens the health of millions of people worldwide, with exposure occurring through contaminated food and water, tobacco use, and industrial activities among other processes.[107] Cadmium contaminates food, water, and tobacco; it is also found in plastics, dyes, and fertilizers.[108] In addition to occupational contact, lead exposure occurs through lead-containing products, including some cosmetics and jewelry, and via inhalation and ingestion from contaminated foods, lead plumbing, lead-based paints, and the largely historical use of leaded gasoline.[109]

Toxic metals/metalloids are linked to multiple acute and chronic adverse health effects through a variety of mechanisms, including oxidative stress, inflammation, and endocrine disruption.[110] Despite similar mechanisms of toxicity, metals/metalloids may uniquely target certain organ systems. With respect to metabolic disease, arsenic and cadmium are noted to disrupt metabolic physiology, promoting the development of insulin resistance and diabetes, with somewhat conflicting evidence regarding their obesogenic properties.[111] Both alone and in combination with other toxic metals, lead is associated with diabetes.[112] These metals are also implicated in other endocrine conditions including thyroid disruption, infertility, and other reproductive disorders.[113–115]

There are important racial disparities in toxic metal/metalloid exposures. For example, lead is a major public health threat in the US, and there is extensive evidence that Black and Hispanic/Latinx families are more highly exposed, especially those who live in low-income areas.[116] Additionally, in utero and postnatal lead biomarkers are higher in Black children.[117] Regions with higher groundwater arsenic levels tend to be home to greater minority populations, especially Hispanics/Latinxs.[118] Exposures also vary across countries as more recently immigrated individuals have higher toxic metal/metalloid levels than individuals who have lived in the US for longer.[119] Lastly, regardless of race/ethnicity, lower SES is associated with increased risk of heavy metal exposures, including lead, cadmium, and arsenic.[120]

Brominated Flame Retardants

Added to consumer products, such as furniture, insulation, plastics, and electronics, flame retardants are synthetic chemicals used to prevent the initiation or spread of fires.[121] The most widely used brominated flame retardants (BFRs) are polybrominated diphenyl ethers (PBDEs) and polybrominated biphenyls. BFRs are persistent pollutants that accumulate in the environment and in human tissue, with contaminated dust the major source of BFR exposures, especially in North America.[122] BFRs are associated with various adverse endocrine health effects, including diabetes, obesity, altered thyroid function, cancer, and reproductive dysfunction.[123]

Studies have shown that lower income individuals and low-income housing residents had higher exposures to PBDEs, especially children.[124,125] There are also

Table 2
Proposed strategies to reduce EDC exposures

Exposure Source	Interventions
Personal and home care	1. Wash hands regularly using fragrance- and antibiotic-free soaps. 2. Regularly clean floors and remove dust using a damp cloth. 3. Eliminate or drastically reduce use of household chemicals, including cleaning supplies, pesticides, and solvents. 4. Choose electrical appliances and lawncare equipment. 5. Forbid smoking indoors. 6. Do not burn trash or yard waste. 7. Read product labels and avoid items containing parabens, bisphenols, and phthalates. 8. Minimize use of products packaged or stored in plastics. 9. Avoid cosmetics with synthetic fragrances, phthalates, or toxic metals. Choose instead those labeled as "no synthetic fragrance," "scented with essential oils," or "phthalate-free." 10. Minimize handling of receipts.
Food and beverages	1. Prioritize eating locally grown fresh or frozen foods. 2. Ensure adequate intake of calcium, iron, and iodine and other essential vitamins and minerals. 3. Consume a diversified diet that is high in fiber. 4. Consult local guidance regarding safe sport fish consumption. 5. Trim fat from meat and skin from fish. Cook meat and fish on a rack to allow fat to drain. 6. Avoid canned, processed, and fast foods. 7. Store food in glass, stainless steel, or porcelain containers. 8. Avoid heating foods in plastic containers. 9. Consider testing your water and using a water filter. 10. Determine whether a lead service line provides water to your home and pursue local programs to remove and replace it.
Travel and transportation	1. Schedule outdoor activities, including exercise, at low traffic times and away from busy roads. 2. Check local air quality and avoid outdoor activities when air pollution levels are high. 3. Pick efficient travel routes that limit time in traffic. 4. Substitute driving with active transportation (walking, cycling, and public transportation). 5. Encourage local school councils to reduce school bus emissions, including "No Idling Zones."
Industrial activities and urban design	1. Advocate for sustainable development, including renewable energy, walkability, bike lanes, and public transit. 2. Promote the expansion of green spaces and tree planting and the elimination of synthetic turf fields and the use of pesticides. 3. Demand transparency in product labeling and access to real-time data on local industrial emissions to empower individual actions.

Adapted from Sargis RM, Heindel JJ, Padmanabhan V. Interventions to Address Environmental Metabolism-Disrupting Chemicals: Changing the Narrative to Empower Action to Restore Metabolic Health. Front Endocrinol (Lausanne). 2019;10:33. Published 2019 Feb 4.

significant gender disparities in BFR exposures. Among young adults in China, women had PBDE levels three-times higher than those of men.[122] Racial/ethnic disparities in BFR exposures are also noted, with Black and Hispanic/Latinx populations having the highest PBDE exposures.[126]

SUMMARY

Multiple social and structural determinants of health undoubtedly contribute to the marked racial/ethnic-, gender-, and socioeconomic-based disparities in endocrine health; however, the contribution of environmental injustice is vastly underappreciated. Indeed, those groups disproportionately burdened by endocrine disorders are often exposed to higher levels of various EDCs, including PCBs, phthalates, bisphenols, OC pesticides, air pollutants, PFASs, toxic metals/metalloids, and BFRs. Furthermore, the contribution of disparate exposures to health disparities is likely underestimated because of a paucity of data examining the adverse effects of combined EDC exposures. As such, health equity requires interventions to address environmental injustice. Such approaches must include a complementary array of individual action and public policy,[127] the latter of which is inadequately used.[128] Based on the Developmental Origins of Health and Disease hypothesis that posits long-term health risks imposed by stressors during sensitive developmental windows (including EDC exposures), it is essential that interventions be targeted to those most vulnerable, including pregnant mothers and infants, among others. However, it is also critical to recognize that EDC exposures and their disproportionate burden on low income and communities of color is a systemic problem for which individual action is insufficient. Rather, policy interventions are required, including robust efforts to identify EDCs before they enter commerce, eliminate EDCs already in use, mitigate contaminated sites, and develop socially just policies that end the discriminatory siting of polluting industries. Vigorously pursued, such efforts have the potential to improve endocrine health equity while reducing the burden of disease for everyone.

CLINICS CARE POINTS

- Health care providers should recognize that EDC exposures may amplify endocrine disease risk and incorporate occupational and environmental history-taking into their practices to identify modifiable patient-specific environmental risk factors.
- Patients should be offered strategies to reduce their exposures to EDCs (**Table 2**).
- Although not yet broadly endorsed, clinicians should follow recommendations of professional organizations and consider measuring EDCs in patients likely to have a history of high-level exposures, as recently recommended for PFASs.
- Health care providers should advocate for incorporation of environmental health into clinical practice guidelines, public policies that promote environmental health, and improved environmental health literacy among the health care workforce and patients.

DISCLOSURE

The views expressed in this article are those of the authors and do not necessarily reflect the position or policy of the Department of Veterans Affairs or the United States government. R.M. Sargis declares he has received honoraria from CVS/Health and the American Medical Forum, neither of which relate to the present study. All other authors declare they have no competing interests. The authors apologize to any authors whose work was omitted because of space limitations.

FUNDING

This work was supported by the National Institutes of Health [R01 ES028879 and P30 ES027792 supporting R.M. Sargis; F30 ES033510 supporting M.C. Weiss; and T32 GM079086 supporting M.C. Weiss and L. Wang via the University of Illinois at Chicago's Medical-Scientist Training Program).

REFERENCES

1. Mikhail N, Wali S, Brown AF. Ethnic disparities in diabetes. Endocrinol Metab Clin North Am 2021;50(3):475–90.
2. Luff MK, Kim J, Tseng CH, et al. Racial/ethnic disparities in thyroid cancer in California, 1999-2017. Am J Surg 2022;225(2):298–303.
3. Morris JR, Plowden TC, Green LJ, et al. Racial and ethnic variation in genetic susceptibility: are disparities in infertility prevalence and outcomes more than Black and White? Reprod Sci 2022;29(7):2081–3.
4. Moore JX, Chaudhary N, Akinyemiju T. metabolic syndrome prevalence by race/ethnicity and sex in the United States, National Health and Nutrition Examination Survey, 1988-2012. Prev Chronic Dis 2017;14:E24.
5. Blanquet M, Legrand A, Pelissier A, et al. Socio-economics status and metabolic syndrome: a meta-analysis. Diabetes Metab Syndr 2019;13(3):1805–12.
6. Bleich SN, Jarlenski MP, Bell CN, et al. Health inequalities: trends, progress, and policy. Annu Rev Public Health 2012;33:7–40.
7. Ruiz D, Becerra M, Jagai JS, et al. Disparities in environmental exposures to endocrine-disrupting chemicals and diabetes risk in vulnerable populations. Diabetes Care 2018;41(1):193–205.
8. Attina TM, Malits J, Naidu M, et al. Racial/ethnic disparities in disease burden and costs related to exposure to endocrine-disrupting chemicals in the United States: an exploratory analysis. J Clin Epidemiol 2019;108:34–43.
9. Ash M, Boyce JK. Racial disparities in pollution exposure and employment at US industrial facilities. Proc Natl Acad Sci U S A 2018;115(42):10636–41.
10. Magliano DJ, Boyko EJ. In: IDF DIABETES ATLAS. 10th ed. Brussels2021.
11. CDC. Centers for Disease Control and Prevention National Diabetes Statistics Report, 2020. . 2020. https://www.cdc.gov/diabetes/pdfs/data/statistics/national-diabetes-statistics-report.pdf.
12. Benjamins MR, Silva A, Saiyed NS, et al. Comparison of all-cause mortality rates and inequities between black and white populations across the 30 most populous US cities. JAMA Netw Open 2021;4(1):e2032086.
13. Volaco A, Cavalcanti AM, Filho RP, et al. Socioeconomic status: the missing link between obesity and diabetes mellitus? Curr Diabetes Rev 2018;14(4):321–6.
14. Ellison-Barnes A, Johnson S, Gudzune K. Trends in obesity prevalence among adults aged 18 through 25 years, 1976-2018. JAMA 2021;326(20):2073–4.
15. Darmon N, Drewnowski A. Contribution of food prices and diet cost to socioeconomic disparities in diet quality and health: a systematic review and analysis. Nutr Rev 2015;73(10):643–60.
16. Lovasi GS, Hutson MA, Guerra M, et al. Built environments and obesity in disadvantaged populations. Epidemiol Rev 2009;31:7–20.

17. Heindel JJ, Howard S, Agay-Shay K, et al. Obesity II: establishing causal links between chemical exposures and obesity. Biochem Pharmacol 2022;199: 115015.
18. Samji NS, Snell PD, Singal AK, et al. Racial disparities in diagnosis and prognosis of nonalcoholic fatty liver disease. Clin Liver Dis 2020;16(2):66–72.
19. Rich NE, Oji S, Mufti AR, et al. Racial and ethnic disparities in nonalcoholic fatty liver disease prevalence, severity, and outcomes in the United States: a systematic review and meta-analysis. Clin Gastroenterol Hepatol 2018;16(2):198–210 e192.
20. Balakrishnan M, Patel P, Dunn-Valadez S, et al. Women have a lower risk of nonalcoholic fatty liver disease but a higher risk of progression vs men: a systematic review and meta-analysis. Clin Gastroenterol Hepatol 2021;19(1): 61–71 e15.
21. Talens M, Tumas N, Lazarus JV, et al. What do we know about inequalities in NAFLD distribution and outcomes? A scoping review. J Clin Med 2021;10(21).
22. The Lancet D, Endocrinology. The untapped potential of the thyroid axis. Lancet Diabetes Endocrinol 2013;1(3):163.
23. Dean DS, Gharib H. Epidemiology of thyroid nodules. Best Pract Res Clin Endocrinol Metab 2008;22(6):901–11.
24. Zhang F, Li Y, Yu X, et al. The relationship and gender disparity between thyroid nodules and metabolic syndrome components based on a recent nationwide cross-sectional study and meta-analysis. Front Endocrinol 2021;12:736972.
25. Iwata AJ, Bhan A, Lahiri S, et al. Incidental thyroid nodules: race/ethnicity disparities and outcomes. Endocr Pract 2018;24(11):941–7.
26. Li Y, Huang D, Wang B, et al. Socioeconomic factors are associated with the prognosis of thyroid cancer. J Cancer 2021;12(9):2507–12.
27. Nnorom SO, Baig H, Akinyemi OA, et al. Persistence of disparity in thyroid cancer survival after adjustments for socioeconomic status and access. Am Surg 2022;88(7):1484–9.
28. McLeod DS, Cooper DS, Ladenson PW, et al. Race/ethnicity and the prevalence of thyrotoxicosis in young Americans. Thyroid 2015;25(6):621–8.
29. Rhee CM, Curhan GC, Alexander EK, et al. Subclinical hypothyroidism and survival: the effects of heart failure and race. J Clin Endocrinol Metab 2013;98(6): 2326–36.
30. Ramnitz MS, Lodish MB. Racial disparities in pubertal development. Semin Reprod Med 2013;31(5):333–9.
31. Velez Edwards DR, Baird DD, Hartmann KE. Association of age at menarche with increasing number of fibroids in a cohort of women who underwent standardized ultrasound assessment. Am J Epidemiol 2013;178(3):426–33.
32. Marsh EE, Al-Hendy A, Kappus D, et al. Burden, prevalence, and treatment of uterine fibroids: a survey of U.S. women. J Womens Health (Larchmt) 2018; 27(11):1359–67.
33. Paramsothy P, Harlow SD, Nan B, et al. Duration of the menopausal transition is longer in women with young age at onset: the multiethnic Study of Women's Health Across the Nation. Menopause 2017;24(2):142–9.
34. Lee I, Vresilovic J, Irfan M, et al. Higher incidence of metabolic syndrome in Black women with polycystic ovary syndrome: a longitudinal study. J Clin Endocrinol Metab 2022;107(4):e1558–67.
35. Walker Z, Rucker L, Owen J, et al. Investigation of racial disparities in semen parameters among white, black, and Asian men. Andrology 2021;9(4):1086–91.

36. Mallidis C, Czerwiec A, Filippi S, et al. Spermatogenic and sperm quality differences in an experimental model of metabolic syndrome and hypogonadal hypogonadism. Reproduction 2011;142(1):63–71.
37. Allen JO, Watkins DC, Chatters L, et al. Cortisol and racial health disparities affecting Black men in later life: evidence from MIDUS II. Am J Men's Health 2019;13(4). 1557988319870969.
38. Steffensen C, Bak AM, Rubeck KZ, et al. Epidemiology of Cushing's syndrome. Neuroendocrinology 2010;92(Suppl 1):1–5.
39. Calhoun DA, Nishizaka MK, Zaman MA, et al. Hyperaldosteronism among black and white subjects with resistant hypertension. Hypertension 2002;40(6):892–6.
40. Gochfeld M, Burger J. Disproportionate exposures in environmental justice and other populations: the importance of outliers. Am J Public Health 2011; 101(Suppl 1):S53–63.
41. James-Todd TM, Chiu YH, Zota AR. Racial/ethnic disparities in environmental endocrine disrupting chemicals and women's reproductive health outcomes: epidemiological examples across the life course. Curr Epidemiol Rep 2016; 3(2):161–80.
42. Belova A, Greco SL, Riederer AM, et al. A method to screen U.S. environmental biomonitoring data for race/ethnicity and income-related disparity. Environ Health 2013;12:114.
43. Street ME, Angelini S, Bernasconi S, et al. Current knowledge on endocrine disrupting chemicals (EDCs) from animal biology to humans, from pregnancy to adulthood: highlights from a national Italian meeting. Int J Mol Sci 2018;19(6).
44. Ribeiro CM, Beserra BTS, Silva NG, et al. Exposure to endocrine-disrupting chemicals and anthropometric measures of obesity: a systematic review and meta-analysis. BMJ Open 2020;10(6):e033509.
45. Wu H, Bertrand KA, Choi AL, et al. Persistent organic pollutants and type 2 diabetes: a prospective analysis in the nurses' health study and meta-analysis. Environ Health Perspect 2013;121(2):153–61.
46. Evangelou E, Ntritsos G, Chondrogiorgi M, et al. Exposure to pesticides and diabetes: a systematic review and meta-analysis. Environ Int 2016;91:60–8.
47. Schulz MC, Sargis RM. Inappropriately sweet: environmental endocrine-disrupting chemicals and the diabetes pandemic. Adv Pharmacol 2021;92: 419–56.
48. Cave M, Appana S, Patel M, et al. Polychlorinated biphenyls, lead, and mercury are associated with liver disease in American adults: NHANES 2003-2004. Environ Health Perspect 2010;118(12):1735–42.
49. Xue J, Liu SV, Zartarian VG, et al. Analysis of NHANES measured blood PCBs in the general US population and application of SHEDS model to identify key exposure factors. J Expo Sci Environ Epidemiol 2014;24(6):615–21.
50. Muennig P, Song X, Payne-Sturges DC, et al. Blood and urine levels of long half-life toxicants by nativity among immigrants to the United States. Sci Total Environ 2011;412-413:109–13.
51. Borrell LN, Factor-Litvak P, Wolff MS, et al. Effect of socioeconomic status on exposures to polychlorinated biphenyls (PCBs) and dichlorodiphenyldichloroethylene (DDE) among pregnant African-American women. Arch Environ Health 2004;59(5):250–5.
52. Helmfrid I, Salihovic S, van Bavel B, et al. Exposure and body burden of polychlorinated biphenyls (PCB) and metals in a historically contaminated community. Environ Int 2015;76:41–8.

53. Schettler T. Human exposure to phthalates via consumer products. Int J Androl 2006;29(1):134–9 [discussion: 181-135].
54. Basso CG, de Araujo-Ramos AT, Martino-Andrade AJ. Exposure to phthalates and female reproductive health: a literature review. Reprod Toxicol 2022;109: 61–79.
55. Radke EG, Glenn BS, Braun JM, et al. Phthalate exposure and female reproductive and developmental outcomes: a systematic review of the human epidemiological evidence. Environ Int 2019;130:104580.
56. Bonde JP, Flachs EM, Rimborg S, et al. The epidemiologic evidence linking prenatal and postnatal exposure to endocrine disrupting chemicals with male reproductive disorders: a systematic review and meta-analysis. Hum Reprod Update 2016;23(1):104–25.
57. Zhang H, Ben Y, Han Y, et al. Phthalate exposure and risk of diabetes mellitus: implications from a systematic review and meta-analysis. Environ Res 2022; 204(Pt B):112109.
58. Egalini F, Marinelli L, Rossi M, et al. Endocrine disrupting chemicals: effects on pituitary, thyroid and adrenal glands. Endocrine 2022;78(3):395–405.
59. Ryva BA, Haggerty DK, Pacyga DC, et al. Determinants of urinary phthalate biomarker concentrations in pre- and perimenopausal women with consideration of race. Environ Res 2022;214(Pt 3):114056.
60. Zota AR, Shamasunder B. The environmental injustice of beauty: framing chemical exposures from beauty products as a health disparities concern. Am J Obstet Gynecol 2017;217(4):418 e411–e418 e416.
61. Han Y, Cheng J, Tang Z, et al. Widespread occurrence of phthalates in popular take-out food containers from China and the implications for human exposure. J Clean Prod 2021;290:125851.
62. Zota AR, Phillips CA, Mitro SD. Recent fast food consumption and bisphenol A and phthalates exposures among the U.S. population in NHANES, 2003-2010. Environ Health Perspect 2016;124(10):1521–8.
63. von Goetz N, Wormuth M, Scheringer M, et al. Bisphenol A: how the most relevant exposure sources contribute to total consumer exposure. Risk Anal 2010; 30(3):473–87.
64. Fenichel P, Chevalier N, Brucker-Davis F. Bisphenol A: an endocrine and metabolic disruptor. Ann Endocrinol 2013;74(3):211–20.
65. Hu Y, Wen S, Yuan D, et al. The association between the environmental endocrine disruptor bisphenol A and polycystic ovary syndrome: a systematic review and meta-analysis. Gynecol Endocrinol 2018;34(5):370–7.
66. Ranciere F, Lyons JG, Loh VH, et al. Bisphenol A and the risk of cardiometabolic disorders: a systematic review with meta-analysis of the epidemiological evidence. Environ Health 2015;14:46.
67. van Woerden I, Bruening M, Montresor-Lopez J, et al. Trends and disparities in urinary BPA concentrations among U.S. emerging adults. Environ Res 2019;176: 108515.
68. Ranjit N, Siefert K, Padmanabhan V. Bisphenol-A and disparities in birth outcomes: a review and directions for future research. J Perinatol 2010;30(1):2–9.
69. Unal ER, Lynn T, Neidich J, et al. Racial disparity in maternal and fetal-cord bisphenol A concentrations. J Perinatol 2012;32(11):844–50.
70. Nelson JW, Scammell MK, Hatch EE, et al. Social disparities in exposures to bisphenol A and polyfluoroalkyl chemicals: a cross-sectional study within NHANES 2003-2006. Environ Health 2012;11:10.

71. Payne-Sturges D, Gee GC. National environmental health measures for minority and low-income populations: tracking social disparities in environmental health. Environ Res 2006;102(2):154–71.
72. Gupta PK. Pesticide exposure: Indian scene. Toxicology 2004;198(1–3):83–90.
73. Jayaraj R, Megha P, Sreedev P. Organochlorine pesticides, their toxic effects on living organisms and their fate in the environment. Interdiscip Toxicol 2016; 9(3–4):90–100.
74. Patterson DG Jr, Wong LY, Turner WE, et al. Levels in the U.S. population of those persistent organic pollutants (2003-2004) included in the Stockholm Convention or in other long range transboundary air pollution agreements. Environ Sci Technol 2009;43(4):1211–8.
75. Sun M, Cao X, Wu Y, et al. Prenatal exposure to endocrine-disrupting chemicals and thyroid function in neonates: a systematic review and meta-analysis. Ecotoxicol Environ Saf 2022;231:113215.
76. Han MA, Kim JH, Song HS. Persistent organic pollutants, pesticides, and the risk of thyroid cancer: systematic review and meta-analysis. Eur J Cancer Prev 2019;28(4):344–9.
77. Turyk ME, Anderson HA, Freels S, et al. Associations of organochlorines with endogenous hormones in male Great Lakes fish consumers and nonconsumers. Environ Res 2006;102(3):299–307.
78. Krstev S, Knutsson A. Occupational risk factors for prostate cancer: a meta-analysis. J Cancer Prev 2019;24(2):91–111.
79. Khanjani N, Hoving JL, Forbes AB, et al. Systematic review and meta-analysis of cyclodiene insecticides and breast cancer. J Environ Sci Health C Environ Carcinog Ecotoxicol Rev 2007;25(1):23–52.
80. Hernandez-Mariano JA, Baltazar-Reyes MC, Salazar-Martinez E, et al. Exposure to the pesticide DDT and risk of diabetes and hypertension: systematic review and meta-analysis of prospective studies. Int J Hyg Environ Health 2022;239: 113865.
81. Lamat H, Sauvant-Rochat MP, Tauveron I, et al. Metabolic syndrome and pesticides: a systematic review and meta-analysis. Environ Pollut 2022;305:119288.
82. Stratakis N, Rock S, La Merrill MA, et al. Prenatal exposure to persistent organic pollutants and childhood obesity: a systematic review and meta-analysis of human studies. Obes Rev 2022;23(Suppl 1):e13383.
83. Roberts EK, Boss J, Mukherjee B, et al. Persistent organic pollutant exposure contributes to Black/White differences in leukocyte telomere length in the National Health and Nutrition Examination Survey. Sci Rep 2022;12(1):19960.
84. Krieger N, Wolff MS, Hiatt RA, et al. Breast cancer and serum organochlorines: a prospective study among white, black, and Asian women. J Natl Cancer Inst 1994;86(8):589–99.
85. Purdue MP, Hoppin JA, Blair A, et al. Occupational exposure to organochlorine insecticides and cancer incidence in the Agricultural Health Study. Int J Cancer 2007;120(3):642–9.
86. Yang BY, Fan S, Thiering E, et al. Ambient air pollution and diabetes: a systematic review and meta-analysis. Environ Res 2020;180:108817.
87. Balti EV, Echouffo-Tcheugui JB, Yako YY, et al. Air pollution and risk of type 2 diabetes mellitus: a systematic review and meta-analysis. Diabetes Res Clin Pract 2014;106(2):161–72.
88. Parasin N, Amnuaylojaroen T, Saokaew S. Effect of air pollution on obesity in children: a systematic review and meta-analysis. Children 2021;8(5).

89. Huang S, Zhang X, Huang J, et al. Ambient air pollution and body weight status in adults: a systematic review and meta-analysis. Environ Pollut 2020;265(Pt A):114999.
90. Sui J, Xia H, Zhao Q, et al. Long-term exposure to fine particulate matter and the risk of chronic liver diseases: a meta-analysis of observational studies. Int J Environ Res Publ Health 2022;19(16).
91. Fathi Najafi T, Latifnejad Roudsari R, Namvar F, et al. Air pollution and quality of sperm: a meta-analysis. Iran Red Crescent Med J 2015;17(4):e26930.
92. Carre J, Gatimel N, Moreau J, et al. Does air pollution play a role in infertility?: a systematic review. Environ Health 2017;16(1):82.
93. Mikati I, Benson AF, Luben TJ, et al. Disparities in distribution of particulate matter emission sources by race and poverty status. Am J Public Health 2018;108(4):480–5.
94. Li Z, Konisky DM, Zirogiannis N. Racial, ethnic, and income disparities in air pollution: a study of excess emissions in Texas. PLoS One 2019;14(8):e0220696.
95. Jerrett M. Global geographies of injustice in traffic-related air pollution exposure. Epidemiology 2009;20(2):231–3.
96. Kodros JK, Bell ML, Dominici F, et al. Unequal airborne exposure to toxic metals associated with race, ethnicity, and segregation in the USA. Nat Commun 2022;13(1):6329.
97. Jones MR, Diez-Roux AV, Hajat A, et al. Race/ethnicity, residential segregation, and exposure to ambient air pollution: the Multi-Ethnic Study of Atherosclerosis (MESA). Am J Public Health 2014;104(11):2130–7.
98. Liu J, Clark LP, Bechle MJ, et al. Disparities in air pollution exposure in the United States by race/ethnicity and income, 1990-2010. Environ Health Perspect 2021;129(12):127005.
99. Jbaily A, Zhou X, Liu J, et al. Air pollution exposure disparities across US population and income groups. Nature 2022;601(7892):228–33.
100. Sunderland EM, Hu XC, Dassuncao C, et al. A review of the pathways of human exposure to poly- and perfluoroalkyl substances (PFASs) and present understanding of health effects. J Expo Sci Environ Epidemiol 2019;29(2):131–47.
101. Armstrong LE, Guo GL. Understanding environmental contaminants' direct effects on non-alcoholic fatty liver disease progression. Curr Environ Health Rep 2019;6(3):95–104.
102. Fraser AJ, Webster TF, Watkins DJ, et al. Polyfluorinated compounds in dust from homes, offices, and vehicles as predictors of concentrations in office workers' serum. Environ Int 2013;60:128–36.
103. Goin DE, Abrahamsson D, Wang M, et al. Disparities in chemical exposures among pregnant women and neonates by socioeconomic and demographic characteristics: a nontargeted approach. Environ Res 2022;215(Pt 1):114158.
104. Ding N, Harlow SD, Batterman S, et al. Longitudinal trends in perfluoroalkyl and polyfluoroalkyl substances among multiethnic midlife women from 1999 to 2011: the Study of Women's Health Across the Nation. Environ Int 2020;135:105381.
105. Santaliz Casiano A, Lee A, Teteh D, et al. Endocrine-disrupting chemicals and breast cancer: disparities in exposure and importance of research inclusivity. Endocrinology 2022;163(5).
106. In: Guidance on PFAS Exposure, Testing, and Clinical Follow-Up. Washington (DC)2022.
107. Jomova K, Jenisova Z, Feszterova M, et al. Arsenic: toxicity, oxidative stress and human disease. J Appl Toxicol 2011;31(2):95–107.

108. Satarug S, Garrett SH. Sens MA, Sens DA. Cadmium, environmental exposure, and health outcomes. Environ Health Perspect 2010;118(2):182–90.
109. Wani AL, Ara A, Usmani JA. Lead toxicity: a review. Interdiscip Toxicol 2015; 8(2):55–64.
110. Rehman K, Fatima F, Waheed I, et al. Prevalence of exposure of heavy metals and their impact on health consequences. J Cell Biochem 2018;119(1):157–84.
111. Haverinen E, Fernandez MF, Mustieles V, et al. Metabolic syndrome and endocrine disrupting chemicals: an overview of exposure and health effects. Int J Environ Res Publ Health 2021;18(24).
112. Wang B, Chen C, Zhang W, et al. Exposure to lead and cadmium is associated with fasting plasma glucose and type 2 diabetes in Chinese adults. Diabetes Metab Res Rev 2022;38(8):e3578.
113. Liang C, Zhang Z, Cao Y, et al. Exposure to multiple toxic metals and polycystic ovary syndrome risk: endocrine disrupting effect from As, Pb and Ba. Sci Total Environ 2022;849:157780.
114. Rattan S, Zhou C, Chiang C, et al. Exposure to endocrine disruptors during adulthood: consequences for female fertility. J Endocrinol 2017;233(3): R109–29.
115. Gustin K, Barman M, Skroder H, et al. Thyroid hormones in relation to toxic metal exposure in pregnancy, and potential interactions with iodine and selenium. Environ Int 2021;157:106869.
116. Lievanos RS, Evans CR, Light R. An intercategorical ecology of lead exposure: complex environmental health vulnerabilities in the Flint water crisis. Int J Environ Res Publ Health 2021;18(5).
117. Cassidy-Bushrow AE, Sitarik AR, Havstad S, et al. Burden of higher lead exposure in African-Americans starts in utero and persists into childhood. Environ Int 2017;108:221–7.
118. Nigra AE, Chen Q, Chillrud SN, et al. Inequalities in public water arsenic concentrations in counties and community water systems across the United States, 2006-2011. Environ Health Perspect 2020;128(12):127001.
119. Fong KC, Heo S, Lim CC, et al. The intersection of immigrant and environmental health: a scoping review of observational population exposure and epidemiologic studies. Environ Health Perspect 2022;130(9):96001.
120. LeBron AMW, Torres IR, Valencia E, et al. The state of public health lead policies: implications for urban health inequities and recommendations for health equity. Int J Environ Res Publ Health 2019;16(6).
121. Wei GL, Li DQ, Zhuo MN, et al. Organophosphorus flame retardants and plasticizers: sources, occurrence, toxicity and human exposure. Environ Pollut 2015; 196:29–46.
122. Li J, Dong Z, Wang Y, et al. Human exposure to brominated flame retardants through dust in different indoor environments: Identifying the sources of concentration differences in hair from men and women. Chemosphere 2018;205:71–9.
123. Kim YR, Harden FA, Toms LM, et al. Health consequences of exposure to brominated flame retardants: a systematic review. Chemosphere 2014;106:1–19.
124. Quiros-Alcala L, Bradman A, Nishioka M, et al. Concentrations and loadings of polybrominated diphenyl ethers in dust from low-income households in California. Environ Int 2011;37(3):592–6.
125. Mehta SS, Applebaum KM, James-Todd T, et al. Associations between sociodemographic characteristics and exposures to PBDEs, OH-PBDEs, PCBs, and PFASs in a diverse, overweight population of pregnant women. J Expo Sci Environ Epidemiol 2020;30(1):42–55.

126. Varshavsky JR, Sen S, Robinson JF, et al. Racial/ethnic and geographic differences in polybrominated diphenyl ether (PBDE) levels across maternal, placental, and fetal tissues during mid-gestation. Sci Rep 2020;10(1):12247.
127. Sargis RM, Heindel JJ, Padmanabhan V. Interventions to address environmental metabolism-disrupting chemicals: changing the narrative to empower action to restore metabolic health. Front Endocrinol 2019;10:33.
128. Shaikh S, Jagai JS, Ashley C, et al. Underutilized and under threat: environmental policy as a tool to address diabetes risk. Curr Diab Rep 2018;18(5):25.
129. Golestanzadeh M, Riahi R, Kelishadi R. Association of exposure to phthalates with cardiometabolic risk factors in children and adolescents: a systematic review and meta-analysis. Environ Sci Pollut Res Int 2019;26(35):35670–86.
130. Ribeiro C, Mendes V, Peleteiro B, et al. Association between the exposure to phthalates and adiposity: a meta-analysis in children and adults. Environ Res 2019;179(Pt A):108780.
131. Sang H, Lee KN, Jung CH, Han K, Koh EH. Association between organochlorine pesticides and nonalcoholic fatty liver disease in the National Health and Nutrition Examination Survey 2003-2004. Sci Rep 2022;12(1):11590.
132. Ghorbani Nejad B, Raeisi T, Janmohammadi P, et al. Mercury exposure and risk of type 2 diabetes: a systematic review and meta-analysis. Int J Clin Pract 2022; 2022:7640227.

UNITED STATES POSTAL SERVICE®

Statement of Ownership, Management, and Circulation (All Periodicals Publications Except Requester Publications)

1. Publication Title	2. Publication Number	3. Filing Date
ENDOCRINOLOGY AND METABOLISM CLINICS OF NORTH AMERICA	000 – 275	9/18/2023
4. Issue Frequency	5. Number of Issues Published Annually	6. Annual Subscription Price
MAR, JUN, SEP, DEC	4	$406.00

7. Complete Mailing Address of Known Office of Publication *(Not printer) (Street, city, county, state, and ZIP+4®)*
ELSEVIER INC.
230 Park Avenue, Suite 800
New York, NY 10169

Contact Person
Malathi Samayan
Telephone *(Include area code)*
91-44-4299-4507

8. Complete Mailing Address of Headquarters or General Business Office of Publisher *(Not printer)*
ELSEVIER INC.
230 Park Avenue, Suite 800
New York, NY 10169

9. Full Names and Complete Mailing Addresses of Publisher, Editor, and Managing Editor *(Do not leave blank)*

Publisher *(Name and complete mailing address)*
Dolores Meloni ELSEVIER INC.
1600 JOHN F KENNEDY BLVD. SUITE 1600
PHILADELPHIA, PA 19103-2899

Editor *(Name and complete mailing address)*
TAYLOR HAYES, ELSEVIER INC.
1600 JOHN F KENNEDY BLVD. SUITE 1600
PHILADELPHIA, PA 19103-2899

Managing Editor *(Name and complete mailing address)*
PATRICK MANLEY, ELSEVIER INC.
1600 JOHN F KENNEDY BLVD. SUITE 1600
PHILADELPHIA, PA 19103-2899

10. Owner *(Do not leave blank. If the publication is owned by a corporation, give the name and address of the corporation immediately followed by the names and addresses of all stockholders owning or holding 1 percent or more of the total amount of stock. If not owned by a corporation, give the names and addresses of the individual owners. If owned by a partnership or other unincorporated firm, give its name and address as well as those of each individual owner. If the publication is published by a nonprofit organization, give its name and address.)*

Full Name	Complete Mailing Address
WHOLLY OWNED SUBSIDIARY OF REED/ELSEVIER, US HOLDINGS	1600 JOHN F KENNEDY BLVD. SUITE 1600 PHILADELPHIA, PA 19103-2899

11. Known Bondholders, Mortgagees, and Other Security Holders Owning or Holding 1 Percent or More of Total Amount of Bonds, Mortgages, or Other Securities. If none, check box → ☐ None

Full Name	Complete Mailing Address
N/A	

12. Tax Status *(For completion by nonprofit organizations authorized to mail at nonprofit rates) (Check one)*
The purpose, function, and nonprofit status of this organization and the exempt status for federal income tax purposes:
☒ Has Not Changed During Preceding 12 Months
☐ Has Changed During Preceding 12 Months *(Publisher must submit explanation of change with this statement)*

13. Publication Title: ENDOCRINOLOGY AND METABOLISM CLINICS OF NORTH AMERICA

14. Issue Date for Circulation Data Below: MAY 2023

15. Extent and Nature of Circulation		Average No. Copies Each Issue During Preceding 12 Months	No. Copies of Single Issue Published Nearest to Filing Date
a. Total Number of Copies *(Net press run)*		167	148
b. Paid Circulation *(By Mail and Outside the Mail)*	(1) Mailed Outside-County Paid Subscriptions Stated on PS Form 3541 (Include paid distribution above nominal rate, advertiser's proof copies, and exchange copies)	100	92
	(2) Mailed In-County Paid Subscriptions Stated on PS Form 3541 *(Include paid distribution above nominal rate, advertiser's proof copies, and exchange copies)*	0	0
	(3) Paid Distribution Outside the Mails Including Sales Through Dealers and Carriers, Street Vendors, Counter Sales, and Other Paid Distribution Outside USPS®	57	46
	(4) Paid Distribution by Other Classes of Mail Through the USPS (e.g., First-Class Mail®)	6	6
c. Total Paid Distribution *[Sum of 15b (1), (2), (3), and (4)]*		163	144
d. Free or Nominal Rate Distribution *(By Mail and Outside the Mail)*	(1) Free or Nominal Rate Outside-County Copies included on PS Form 3541	3	3
	(2) Free or Nominal Rate In-County Copies Included on PS Form 3541	0	0
	(3) Free or Nominal Rate Copies Mailed at Other Classes Through the USPS (e.g., First-Class Mail)	0	0
	(4) Free or Nominal Rate Distribution Outside the Mail *(Carriers or other means)*	1	1
e. Total Free or Nominal Rate Distribution *(Sum of 15d (1), (2), (3) and (4))*		4	4
f. Total Distribution *(Sum of 15c and 15e)*		167	148
g. Copies not Distributed *(See Instructions to Publishers #4 (page #3))*		0	0
h. Total *(Sum of 15f and g)*		167	148
i. Percent Paid *(15c divided by 15f times 100)*		97.6%	97.3%

* If you are claiming electronic copies, go to line 16 on page 3. If you are not claiming electronic copies, skip to line 17 on page 3.

16. Electronic Copy Circulation	Average No. Copies Each Issue During Preceding 12 Months	No. Copies of Single Issue Published Nearest to Filing Date
a. Paid Electronic Copies		
b. Total Paid Print Copies (Line 15c) + Paid Electronic Copies (Line 16a)		
c. Total Print Distribution (Line 15f) + Paid Electronic Copies (Line 16a)		
d. Percent Paid (Both Print & Electronic Copies) (16b divided by 16c × 100)		

☒ **I certify that 50% of all my distributed copies (electronic and print) are paid above a nominal price.**

17. Publication of Statement of Ownership
☒ If the publication is a general publication, publication of this statement is required. Will be printed in the DECEMBER 2023 issue of this publication. ☐ Publication not required.

18. Signature and Title of Editor, Publisher, Business Manager, or Owner
Malathi Samayan - Distribution Controller — *Malathi Samayan* — Date: 9/18/2023

I certify that all information furnished on this form is true and complete. I understand that anyone who furnishes false or misleading information on this form or who omits material or information requested on the form may be subject to criminal sanctions (including fines and imprisonment) and/or civil sanctions (including civil penalties).

Printed and bound by CPI Group (UK) Ltd, Croydon, CR0 4YY
08/05/2025
01864750-0008